MW01258232

ĀYURVEDIC YOGA

3 APPROACHES TO TEACHING ĀYURVEDIC YOGA

MONA L. WARNER

This book is not intended as a substitute for the medical advice of physicians. The reader should regularly consult a physician in matters relating to his/her health and particularly with respect to any symptoms that may require diagnosis or medical attention.

Publishing services provided by Archangel Ink

ISBN-13: 978-1-9994272-0-7

To the teachings of Yoga—
with gratitude for giving me my life back.

To the teachings of Āyurveda—
with gratitude for giving me my health back.

CONTENTS

DISCLAIMERS

Dear Reader,

I wanted to bring a few things into your awareness as you dive deeper into this book.

1. This book is not a substitute for medical advice. Although both Yoga and Āyurveda are wonderful in supporting and maintaining health, if you have a health concern, injury, illness, or disease, please refer to a medical or health care practitioner. One of the benefits of living at this time is the availability of health care options—please use all the tools at your disposal to support you.

2. In writing this book for yoga teachers I made two overarching assumptions. The first one being that ***ahiṃsā*** (non-harming, love, reverence, and compassion for all beings) is considered at all times in all offerings. From this comes the second assumption, that you, a yoga teacher, understand that ***not all techniques are appropriate for all students***; this refers to *āsana* (postures), *prāṇāyāma* (breath work), *dhyāna* (meditation), *mantra* (sacred sound), *mudrā* (sacred gestures), and *kriyā* (cleansing techniques). Please remember that all techniques have cautions and some have contraindications. If you are unsure about the cautions and contraindications of any technique, please refer to your teacher, or you can refer to the *Resources for Cautions and Contraindications* at the end of this book.

3. I write about and teach Āyurveda and Yoga using the same lens. Through the process of reviewing and editing this book in preparation for publishing, it was pointed out to me that I teach, and therefore write, with a strong bent toward what is now referred to as *trauma-informed* yoga. I work with a lot of students who have chronic pain and trauma in their history—both diagnosed and undiagnosed trauma. This is my truth. I share this so that as you read through the content, you can keep in mind that this book is written with a trauma-informed lens. I encourage you to consider what lenses you teach through and how you would use the principles presented in this book to work with your own students in their own context. It is so very important to meet our students where they are.

4. Sanskrit. Two things happened here. First, we used the 2016 Style Guide for the *Yoga Samachar* as a guideline for how to note and work with the Sanskrit. In this guide, since yoga as a general team was not capitalized or italicized, we followed the same convention for guṇa, doṣa, and cakra. We made the same decision about Āyurveda.

Second, I have used diacritical marks for the Sanskrit in this book. I used Nicolai Bachman's two books as a reference:

- *The Language of Yoga*. Boulder CO: Sounds True, 2004.
- *The Language of Āyurveda*. Canada: Trafford, 2005.

I also used the Internet a little too. That said, any errors in nomenclature or diacritical marks are mine.

I do not intend this book to be a Sanskrit primer, so if you're looking to dive deeper here, please work with Nicolai Bachman or his wonderful books.

The diacritics used in this book are as follows:

1. ḍ → sounds like dove
2. ḥ → is described as "out breath." This means that one "expires" (out breath) the sound of the vowel that comes before the ḥ. For example, *śantiḥ* is pronounced "shantihi."
3. ṭ → sounds like tub
4. ṃ → sounds like hum
5. ṇ → sounds like tint, with tongue touching the teeth
6. ṛ → sounds like rim
7. ṣ → sounds like schnapps
8. ś Ś → sounds like shut
9. ā Ā → sounds like tar or father, held for 2 beats
10. ī → sounds like week or need, held for 2 beats
11. ū → sounds like fool or mood, held for 2 beats
12. ṅ → sounds like sing
13. ñ → sounds like inch
14. c with no "h" → sounds like church
15. c with an "h" → sounds like much honey

There is much more to linguistics and Sanskrit; however, this should be enough to help you navigate this book.

I wrote this book to share approaches around teaching

Āyurvedic Yoga, based in my experience and exploration. My intention is to support yoga teachers in their exploration of Āyurvedic Yoga. Through this process it was mentioned that a collaborative peer reviewed “textbook of Āyurvedic Yoga” could be useful. If you believe that our community would benefit from this kind of textbook, please let me know. I am happy to plan for a second edition to this book that could become a more formal textbook.

I won’t keep you any longer. Enjoy exploring Āyurvedic Yoga!

Big love,
m xo

NOTE FROM THE AUTHOR

Dear reader,

Namaste!

Thank you so much for picking up this book and giving Āyurvedic Yoga a try! I wrote this with much humility. This book was created out of my desire to have had a guide like this when I started studying Āyurvedic Yoga. I am most grateful to you for reading it.

Integrating Yoga and Āyurveda

As I was exploring how to mix Yoga and Āyurveda, I realized that combining two separate and distinct sciences holds quite a challenge. In my search, I learned there weren't many resources available to help me figure out how to blend Yoga and Āyurveda together while maintaining the integrity of each distinct science. Plus, I needed the practices to be straightforward enough for my students to understand. Some of my students were new to Yoga, and others were new to Āyurveda. The resources I did find were helpful and thoughtfully written; however, they were too complex for my students. If I'm being completely honest, some of these writings were over my head too.

A few years ago, I had an interesting experience at a wellness shop where I live in Kingston, Canada. I was chatting with one of the owners, who is a friend of mine, and she introduced me to a young woman who was considering moving to

Kingston to launch her business—a modality that blended Western nutrition, Yogic Cakra theory, Āyurveda, and Traditional Chinese Medicine. With interest and curiosity, I asked this young woman how long she had been studying these modalities.

"I took a six-month online course," she said.

Reconciling Yoga, Āyurveda, and Western nutrition requires education and practice to deeply understand any one of these modalities. Through my dozen years of Yin Yoga practice and study, I now have a very basic understanding of Traditional Chinese Medicine, another huge modality. I am also aware that TCM is different from Āyurveda right down to the fundamentals—they have a different set of five elements. In TCM, it is Wood, Fire, Earth, Metal, and Water, while the Vedic traditions use Ether, Air, Fire, Water, and Earth. At their very essence, they're different. I was genuinely curious how this woman was able to reconcile the fundamental differences and then add all the other information in a way that maintained the integrity—and therefore the potency—of each science.

In my experience, one needs many years of dedicated study in any science to develop proficiency and a deep understanding of the material. Each science has its own potency and power. If we mix too many things together, we risk diluting them, which waters down their medicinal and healing effects. The greater the dilution, the less potent it is.

Something inside me responded strongly to that conversation with the young woman. I believe that blending Yoga and Āyurveda by simply skimming the surface doesn't do justice to the teachings of either science. The challenge of blending modalities is to maintain the potency, power, and integrity of each as you combine them together. Each of these Vedic sciences incorporates thousands of years of wisdom, practice, and experience.

We know Yoga has been practiced for thousands of years as the science of self-realization. Not only is the science vast, but there are also a variety of approaches to its practice: maybe you're refining through the emotional body (*Bhakti* Yoga), the intellect (*Jñāna* Yoga), your day-to-day actions (Karma Yoga), the physical body (*Haṭha* Yoga), or through meditation (*Rāja* Yoga).

Āyurveda is the oldest continuously practiced medical science in the world. We have evidence of its practice dating back five thousand years! This is a deep and rich study of natural rhythms for healing the human being (all beings, actually) in body and mind. Even in the Āyurvedic context, there are different approaches to the practice and implementation of the tools, right down to which classical text you hold as authoritative for your practice.

We have these two modalities, each of them brilliant in their own right. One is a medical science, and one is a science of self-realization. I'm all for blending them together—*as long as* we remember each of them individually and bring them together in a way that honours each set of teachings. For those of us who want to blend these Vedic sciences, we have one pretty cool thing on our side: Āyurveda uses Yoga as part of its treatment.

Given this overlap, it's not far-fetched that we blend them. When Āyurveda uses Yoga in the treatment of a disease, it's called Yoga Therapy. It is different from a group Yoga class. And although there may be therapeutic benefits to doing Yoga in general, generalized Yoga is not Yoga Therapy. Most of us facilitate a group of folks who are coming together to have a Yoga experience; and in an Āyurvedic Yoga class, the choice of postures, breath work, meditations, tone of voice, and focal points are being influenced by the lens of Āyurveda.

I believe integrating Āyurveda into Yoga classes creates more potency in the Yoga tools and techniques. I hope you can see how merging two sciences, each representing thousands of years of wisdom, can create either the most potent medicine or the biggest mess ever. I deeply want to help other teachers create powerful medicine with Yoga. Āyurvedic Yoga is medicine not only for us, but for our students as well.

The Power of Āyurvedic Yoga

The analogy I use with my students is this: Āyurveda describes the human body-mind as a series of channels, like the pipes that form the plumbing in your house. Some of these channels have food and wastes flowing through them; others have energy and emotions flowing through them; and still others have thoughts, ideas, and inspirations flowing through them. We are healthy when our channels are strong and clear, when things can flow freely through the channels—meaning they can flow freely in and flow freely out. The reality of life is that things happen to disrupt this free flow. Sometimes stuff gets stuck in the channels: the sticky, gooey residue of undigested food, emotions, experiences, and thoughts, known as *āma*. *Āma* clogs our pipes. At other times, the pipes can rust, weaken, or spring leaks. Any of these things can disrupt the flow, which disrupts our sense of well-being.

Enter Yoga and Āyurveda. One way of looking at Yoga and Āyurveda, and understanding their healing potential, is to recognize that a consistent and dedicated practice of Yoga and Āyurveda does two things:

1. it removes clogs from our pipes (I call this *pipe banging*), and
2. it strengthens the pipes so the whole system has more integrity and can handle greater flow.

This is what Yoga and Āyurveda have done for me. I had major clogs, rust, and weakness in my pipes. The way this manifested in my experience was through regular seizures (both grand mal and petit mal), digestive issues, anxiety, depression, and depletion. Yoga helped tremendously; however, when I added the layer of Āyurveda to my life, it brought me to a state of health and clarity I did not know existed. I joke that I'm a poster child for all the amazing things Yoga and Āyurveda can offer a human being willing to practice. Yet, I am no more special or gifted than any other human on this planet. This is why I am so passionate about sharing these teachings—and doing it in a way that maintains the integrity and healing potential of each science. Diluted, we might as well be doing aerobics, which is a healthy thing for some people, but it's not going to heal your nerves, guts, and heart the way Yoga and Āyurveda can.

Approaches to Āyurvedic Yoga

Approach #1: Guṇa Yoga

The language of Āyurveda is simple and accessible. This fundamental language is called the ***Guṇas***, which translates to "quality, attribute, or characteristic." These refer to the qualities of nature. I believe we can integrate Āyurveda into Yoga in a way that will support our understanding of doṣa and all other Āyurvedic concepts through **Guṇa Yoga**,[1] Yoga based in the Āyurvedic qualities of nature.

Focusing on one or two guṇas (qualities) per class, you can adapt your approach to *āsana* (postures), *prāṇāyāma* (breath work), *dhyāna* (meditation), *mantra* (sacred sound), and *mudrā* (gestures) so that everything you do in that class helps to balance the qualities of nature you are focusing on. It is so simple that 90% of my students understand the concept immediately. In a way, you could say the language of Āyurveda (the guṇas) creates a theme, and this quality guides all the techniques that you choose, how you teach them, and so on. Maybe it's hot out, so we use all these different Yoga techniques to cool down. Maybe life feels hard, so we use Yoga practices to cultivate softness. Maybe we feel overwhelmed, so we use Yoga practices to stabilize. I learned this simple approach works really well for me and for my students.

I began to explore Guṇa Yoga with the qualities I could easily figure out, like hot and cold. I started with what I knew, then I figured out how to practice and teach the Yoga techniques

1 A big thanks to Laurel for the name. It was her idea to call it "Guṇa Yoga."

to cultivate that one quality in my students' embodied experience. How do we breathe in a way that increases stability? How do we breathe in a way that increases warmth? How do we breathe in a way that increases a sense of lightness in the body? How do we practice the poses to cultivate a particular quality? How do we meditate to cultivate those same energies?

Using the Āyurvedic lens with the Yoga tools adds an opportunity for the students to understand their connection to nature better. It allows them to get to know themselves and realize their own patterns and rhythms.

My students got it; pretty much everyone understands hot and cold, heavy and light, hard and soft, even if they don't know their *doṣa*. I knew it was working when students came to class and said, "Okay, it's really cold outside, so we need to do a warming practice. And I'm feeling all over the place, so we have to stabilize and simplify at the same time." Bingo! My students were *speaking to me* in Āyurveda talk. That was when I realized I had found a great approach because the students really got it!

With the foundational language of Āyurveda in place, we could grow into doṣas. Students understood where we were going and what we were doing.

Approach #2: Doṣa Yoga

Most of the available resources use a doṣa-based (bio-psychological constitution) approach. They state, for example, that if you are *vāta doṣa* (air and ether predominant) then you should do Tree pose, Mountain pose, and many seated poses.

If you are *pitta* doṣa (fire and water predominant) then you should do Triangle pose, lots of twists, and Shoulderstand. If you are *kapha doṣa* (water and earth predominant), you practice Bow pose, Headstand, and many Sun Salutations.

I love Doṣa Yoga; however, I struggled with applying it in group classes because they were filled with students of many different doṣas. Also, most of my students had no idea what doṣa was, never mind what *their* doṣa was. It took me many years to really understand the concept of doṣa—and twelve years to figure out my own doṣa!

When I attended the Kripalu School of Āyurveda (I LOVE YOU, KSA!)[2], we were taught that everyone embodies all three doṣas in some capacity. With that theory, their approach was different than the books I had read. They taught us that balancing a doṣa doesn't have to be posture specific, it can be approach specific. By changing the tone of voice, pace of the class, and focal point, we were able to use all the poses to balance all the doṣas. It's a wonderful approach! As someone with a lot of *vāta* doṣa, I still want to practice twists and headstands … and now I understand how to approach my practice, so I can do these postures without going out of balance. They also taught us to look beyond the individuals in a class. Yoga teachers know it's hard to give privates to thirty people all at the same time. Yet we can recognize and teach to the doṣa of the season, which is the common thread for all of us. This is one way to bring Yoga and Āyurveda together:

---

2 The programs and trainings I took were amazing! I have been blessed with gifted teachers. To each of you, I bow deeply with more gratitude than I have the ability to express.

share the teachings of Āyurveda using the tools of Yoga with our mixed-student groups.

These are the two main approaches I have found, and both are based on a deep understanding of the doṣas. Not everyone has that level of understanding. For the first approach, not all students know their constitution, so how do they know what to practice? It took me twelve years to figure out my doṣa, and I was trying! I can only imagine that for someone who is new to this, it might take a while to figure things out. For the second approach, what if a season doesn't fit cleanly into a doṣa? What if there's overlap and even contradiction in the weather patterns? Then what do we teach?

This is why I believe Guṇa Yoga comes before Doṣa Yoga. Guṇas support us to integrate Āyurveda into Yoga in a way that will support our understanding of doṣa, and all the other Āyurvedic concepts too.

Approach #3: Special Topics in Āyurveda

After years of exploring Guṇa Yoga, I got creative in a third way. There are other concepts unique to the Āyurvedic teachings, and you can build classes around these ideas. In order to do this, you still need to understand the language, the guṇas. From there, it grows and evolves on its own … at least it does for me. I suspect it will do the same for you. You can read more about these ideas in the third section of this book.

Goals of This Book

I write this book for Yoga teachers, like myself, who recognize that Āyurveda is extremely useful as a co-practice to Yoga. If you're a practicing yogi, having some sort of Āyurvedic practice to support you will help you stay healthy, so you can focus on your Yoga. In the Yoga Sūtras, Patañjali describes nine obstacles to the practice of Yoga, the first one being disease, and the goal of Āyurveda, according to Caraka[3], is to maintain the health of the healthy person. Without health, yogis are limited in the progress they can make on their path. What a great connection between Yoga and Āyurveda!

For you to teach Āyurvedic Yoga to your students, you need to practice, experience, and develop your understanding of how these fit together and what the effects are. In this book, I'm going to give you a few maps. However, these are no substitute for your own practice and experience. Until you have this wisdom in your bones, it's going to be a challenge to share it with your students. I believe one of the biggest mistakes we make as Yoga teachers is sharing things with our students that we have not fully digested.[4]

I'm also very aware there are students who are studying and practicing at a deep level without ever becoming Yoga teachers themselves. They might also want to use this book as a way of exploring how to enhance their Yoga practice by applying and engaging in an exploration of the Āyurvedic lens

3 Caraka is the author of one of the main classical *Āyurvedic* texts.

4 I call it "spewing *āma*." Those of you with a background in *Āyurveda* know exactly what I'm talking about!

to go along with their Yoga toolkit. To me this makes sense because Yoga teachers, hopefully, are also Yoga students.

This book is not for Āyurvedis to learn Yoga. Those who want to learn Yoga techniques and how to teach them need to find a Yoga teacher training program. This book assumes a basic Yoga teacher level of knowledge and teaching experience (for example a 200-hr level YTT), so I'm not going to cover that in the content.

As much as I wish this book had existed when I was trying to figure out how to blend Yoga and Āyurveda skilfully, I am grateful for the beautiful and brilliant exploration this journey has gifted me. It's a journey I am still actively engaged in. I appreciate all of it. Now that I'm practicing Āyurvedic Yoga, I believe what I have learned is of value to other teachers who want to blend Yoga and Āyurveda with integrity.

My hope is that by giving you multiple approaches, you will have choices. I hope to empower you to choose what makes the most sense for you and your students, given the context you find yourselves in. I also hope this book supports your exploration of how to blend Āyurveda and Yoga together in a skilful way—one that allows you to turn Yoga into Āyurvedic medicine for yourself and your students.

Enjoy!
m, xo

SECTION 1

GUṆA YOGA

INTRODUCTION TO THE GUṆAS: THE LANGUAGE OF ĀYURVEDA

Welcome to the section on the guṇas of Āyurveda. The Sanskrit word *guṇa* translates to "characteristic, attribute, or quality." This is the core concept in this book. It is the language of Āyurveda and a foundational concept in all Āyurvedic teachings. When you go to Āyurveda school, the first thing you learn is the 10 pairs of opposites, the 20 qualities that are inherent in all things in *prakṛti* (the world of form). Āyurveda uses the language of the guṇas to describe absolutely everything in nature and the entire universe! For this reason, we need to learn and understand the guṇas. If Yoga teachers can figure this part out, the rest of Āyurveda is straightforward.

Personally, this is the part of Āyurveda I found the most challenging. It asked me to reorganize how I thought about the world. Without understanding guṇas, we can't understand doṣas (bio-psychological constitution) or other Āyurvedic concepts. Neither can we balance anything.

Āyurveda works, like all sciences, by applying or removing a particular stimulus to find balance. Understanding the guṇas allows us to narrow the possibilities so that what we try is not a shot in the dark. When you understand how the laws of nature work, it's easier to apply a stimulus that gives you the response you're looking for.

When we understand the guṇas and how the pairs of opposites work, we know how to find balance. We know exactly what we're looking for, and we know which stimulus to apply to move in the direction of the desired result. This is why understanding the guṇas is critical to successfully using Yoga to bring ourselves (and our students) into balance. This is how Āyurveda works.

Another reason the language of Āyurveda is important, and something I love about this concept, is when you're looking at the world through the lens of the guṇas, there's no judgment. For example, ask a student to check in with the temperature of their body: "Do you feel hot, or do you feel cold?" Neither response—hot or cold—is good or bad. They simply are. Maybe today you're feeling cold; maybe today you're feeling warm. It is what it is. We can take the often-imposed layer of judgment, guilt, shame, and critical mind-set right out of play. This allows us to use Yoga the way it was designed, as a science of self-inquiry and self-realization. By using a language that is inherently non-critical, we develop the capacity to observe ourselves in a way that is compassionate (*ahiṃsā*) and real (*satya*). Now we're getting somewhere.

The brilliance of blending Yoga and Āyurveda is in using the *language of Āyurveda* to inform our choice of *techniques (and the delivery) of Yoga*. We can give our students a whole language with which to observe themselves and their world, one that is compassionate and real, free from critical judgment, guilt, shame, blame, and weirdness. I love this idea of Guṇa Yoga—the Yoga of the qualities of nature.

Hopefully you are beginning to understand, based on this initial idea of the language of Āyurveda, that this book isn't going to give you a class plan—because you're going to *plan the same classes you've always planned.* What's going to change when you learn about these qualities is the delivery of the material and the WHY behind your choices.

First, you begin to embody the qualities you need in order to bring balance to your own system. From there, you can invite and guide your students to do the same thing. If you're a *Vinyāsa* teacher, you're still going to teach *Vinyāsa*. And if you're a Gentle teacher, you're still going to teach Gentle Yoga. You will simply add this dimension of understanding rooted in the Āyurvedic teachings.

The language of Āyurveda is straightforward, making it simple enough to teach to all students. As you impart this language, your students will understand themselves better, and they will understand how they fit into the greater context of nature and life.

The guṇas are a very specific language. With time and practice, your ability to work with this language will evolve and broaden. My intention is to give you a solid starting point. From there, you will go where you need to.

I also want to share that it took me a few years to figure out Guṇa Yoga. There was a lot of trial and error. There are some guṇas I'm more comfortable working with than others. Even with many years of teaching Yoga and studying Āyurveda, it is still a work in progress. This is what I love about this exploration! Many years into teaching Yoga, I'm still developing a more nuanced understanding of how to use the tools more skilfully.[5]

Let's get to the guṇas!

5 To write this section of the book, I collaborated with two dear friends, Veronica and Gummo. I am eternally grateful for their support because where I got stuck, they helped me get unstuck. We opened up one can of worms, after can of worms, after can of worms for you. I hope you like worms.

THE GUṆAS:
THE PAIRS OF OPPOSITES

The table below outlines the guṇas in fixed sets known as "the pairs of opposites."[6] Knowing the guṇas along with their pairing is key to using them skilfully, as we will discover. I've included the Sanskrit translation for those of you who, like myself, enjoy the study and use of Sanskrit as part of the practice.

	Continuum	Building & nourishing (*Brmhana*)	Reducing & lightening (*Langhana*)
1	Weight	Heavy (*Guru*)	Light (*Laghu*)
2	Intensity	Slow or Dull (*Manda*)	Sharp or Penetrating (*Tīkṣṇa*)
3	Temperature	Cold (*Hima or Śīta*)	Hot (*Uṣṇa*)
4	Emollience	Oily or Unctuous (*Snigdha or Sneha*)	Dry (*Rūkṣa*)
5	Texture	Smooth (Ślakṣṇa)	Rough (*Khara*)
6	Viscosity	Dense or Thick or Solid (*Sāndra*)	Liquid or Diluted (*Drava*)
7	Compressibility	Soft (*Mṛdu*)	Hard (*Kaṭhina*)
8	Fluidity	Stable (*Sthira*)	Mobile or Unstable (*Cala*)
9	Density	Gross or Big or Obvious (*Sthūla*)	Subtle (*Sūkṣma*)
10	Adhesion	Cloudy or Slimy Sticky (*Picchila*)	Clear (*Viśada*)

6 From the *Aṣṭāṅga Hṛdayam, Sūtrasthāna* 1.18.

Are you curious about why we have these pairs of opposites? There are a few reasons. One is because we recognize that those opposites are connected. My teacher, Dr. Claudia Welch, explains them as the "yin and yang of Āyurveda." On one end, you've got one quality, and on the other end, you have the opposite quality, and yet one doesn't exist without the other. You can't tell if something is light unless you compare it to something heavy. And the light object, when compared to something else, might be the heavier of the two. Here's an example: if I take my cat, who's 20 pounds,[7] and I compare her to my dog, who's 60 pounds, then we would describe the cat as light. However, if I compare my cat to a piece of paper from my printer, now the cat is heavy.

The qualities are not about a fixed point, and our understanding and interpretation of them is relative to our experience. All the qualities are relative to your own internal sense of balance. When we're working with the guṇas in class and we invite our students to check in ("Do you feel hot or cold today?"), it's an internal check. Either they feel warmer than before, in which case they feel warm or hot, or they feel colder than before, in which case they feel cool or cold. There's even a third option: maybe they can't tell. I interpret this to mean they've found their balance point in the middle of the pair of opposites.

Another aspect of this is what feels hot or warming for me, as someone who tends to run cold, might be different from someone who runs hot. Their starting point on the continuum is different from mine. Everyone's pendulum of balance is different. This is why one regimen does not work for everyone.

7 Yes, I recognize that my cat is larger than average.

We're all different in terms of which qualities we embody, and therefore what we need in order to find balance.

Like Increases Like[8]

Understanding these pairs of opposites is important because this is how we're going to bring balance into the system. If we (ourselves, our students, the environment, nature) are on one end of the continuum, this means the pendulum of balance has swung in one direction. In Āyurveda, we learn that applying the same quality to itself increases that quality.

The example I give my students when I introduce this concept is: "If you're feeling warm, and I offer you a cup of hot tea and wrap you in a blanket and turn up the heat by 10 degrees, what's going to happen?" And everybody looks at me and says, "I'm going to get warmer and be way too hot." And I say, "That's right because *like increases like*." When we apply the same quality to a quality that already exists, we are going to have more of that quality. Like increases like.

Opposites Balance[9]

Then I give the opposite scenario: if you're feeling too warm, and I give you a cup of iced tea and open the window and turn on the fan and get a little breeze going and invite you to take off your socks and your hat and coat, then what happens? And they say, "Then we cool down and we feel better." Applying the opposite quality brings things back into the middle, back into balance.

---

8 From the *Aṣṭāṅga Hṛdayam, Sūtrasthāna* 1.14.1.

9 From the *Aṣṭāṅga Hṛdayam, Sūtrasthāna* 1.14.1.

These pairs of opposites are really important because they give us a language with which to express our felt experience, and they also give us a way to bring balance into our systems.

A question that arises frequently is: "Increasing or reducing?" By this I mean if someone is too cold, do I add heat or do I remove cold? It's a great question. The answer is: It depends. If the option to remove the root cause of suffering (excess cold) exists, then remove the root cause. If the root cause cannot be determined, or you cannot remove it (e.g., being at the North Pole—you can't change the weather), then applying the opposite (hot quality) is what will bring balance.

Guṇa Yoga

The language of the guṇas is powerful, given the scope and depth of what you can describe using these terms. In Āyurveda school we are asked to figure out which qualities are present in our food and lifestyle and in ourselves. We can do the same thing with Yoga. We can either: figure out how to teach a technique to increase one quality or the other, or figure out which techniques fit on which side of the continuum. This was a game-changing moment for me in terms of teaching Āyurvedic Yoga. Āyurveda's guṇas gave me a universal language that translated Yoga in a simple and accessible way.

Let's use *prāṇāyāma* (breath work) as an example. We'll also keep working with the hot and cold qualities because these are straightforward. If we look at *Ujjāyī Prāṇāyāma* (Victorious or Ocean Sounding Breath), what does it do? It warms the body, which means it increases the hot quality. If we apply this technique in the middle of summer to a student having hot flashes, what will the result be? They will get warmer. Then we can ask ourselves (or ask them) if practicing *ujjāyī prāṇāyāma* makes sense, given their context of hot flashes? In all honesty, it depends. There are no right or wrong answers, only opportunities to understand the laws of karma. Yet if they want to stop the hot flashes in the middle of summer, choosing *ujjāyī* isn't going to help them with their cause. They will find more balance by using a cooling breath, like the *Simha Prāṇāyāma* (Lion's Breath), Sighing Breath, *Śītalī*, or *Śītakarī Prāṇāyāma*, which are cooling breaths.[10] That said, they might choose to keep *ujjāyī*, but now they're aware it could be contributing to their menopausal overheating discomfort.

We have now opened a portal into awesomeness. When we teach our students about the qualities and pairs of opposites, we have given them a language and a set of tools they can use to self-regulate and achieve balance. Now when someone is having a hot flash, they know how to breathe (or how not to breathe) in order to change their internal qualities. They can learn how to apply a stimulus that gives them the response they need so they can find balance and feel better. I can't think of anything more awesome.

In this next section, I will describe each quality, its opposite, and how the Yoga techniques fit in with the guṇas.

I love dictionaries and definitions, so I've included the dictionary definition[11] of each guṇa because it's fascinating to think of these guṇas in as many ways as possible.

---

10 Do you recognize the Sanskrit connection from the guṇa chart? *Śīta* means cold.

11 The Google Dictionary is the source of these definitions.

In the description of each quality, I'll discuss how each guṇa shows up in the environment or nature, the body, and the mind and emotions. Then I'll discuss when you might want to work with each guṇa, and how to cultivate that quality in a Yoga context in terms of pace, language and approach, *āsana* (postures), *prāṇāyāma* (breath work), *dhyāna* (meditation), *mantra* (sacred sound), *mudrā* (gestures), and the integration of the practice.[12]

12 A lot of folks refer to this part of the practice as "*Śavāsana*." Technically *Śavāsana* (Corpse) is a pose, and the process of the integration of the practice can happen successfully (even more so, one might argue) in a variety of poses. Here, I am not referring to a pose but the process of absorption and integration of the whole practice.

CHAPTER 1

WEIGHT: HEAVY AND LIGHT

A. HEAVY GUṆA

Environment / Nature

In nature, the heavy quality is related to the earth element. Earth is the heaviest of the five elements in Vedic Science. The dictionary defines *heavy* as "of great weight; difficult to lift or move" and "needing much physical effort."[13]

We find heaviness in the mountains, the ocean,[14] gravity, and soil. Elephants, trucks, buildings, bowling balls, metals, and trains are all heavy.

In the weather, heaviness manifests as wet snow,[15] mud, big rainfalls, and in dense clouds.[16]

Body

In the body, we see heavy bones, heavy muscles, and a larger frame or skeleton. If there is an excess of the heavy quality, people become overweight. Foods that have the heavy quality are very nourishing, which means they are excellent

13 "Heavy," Google, accessed March 2018, https://www.google.ca/search?q=Dictionary.

14 Have you carried a 10L bottle of water? Can you imagine the weight of an ocean?

15 If you've ever shovelled it, you know how heavy this is!

16 Often described as a "heavy sky."

for building tissues in the body. Culturally, we tend to think that being heavy or overweight is "bad." We add a value judgment that is not inherently there, and we miss the other aspect, which is that nourishment is necessary. We want to cultivate enough heaviness that we're feeling nourished but not so much that we end up with excess. We are looking for our balance point even within the one quality.

Heaviness can manifest in a deep voice. Folks who embody heaviness feel grounded, centered, and stable. This is neat because stability is one of the other qualities in our list. We will see that sometimes the qualities work together and are not mutually exclusive. There is definitely interconnection between the different guṇas.

The heavy quality manifests as slow digestion or slow metabolism, which means it takes a long time for food to digest. Slow digestion also happens if you eat too much heavy food, regardless of the nature of your digestion. Examples of heavy foods include meats potatoes, dairy, and in an extreme form as a deep-fried cheesesteak hoagie.[17]

Mind and Emotions

We need enough of the heavy quality in order to fall asleep at night, which is super important, as sleep is one of Āyurveda's three pillars of health. It also manifests as deep thoughts. Where there's excess heaviness in the mind, one might feel tired, depressed, or like the world is too heavy.[18]

---

17 Which I suspect is the heaviest food ever created.

18 As the expression goes, "Carrying the weight of the world on our shoulders."

Cultivating the HEAVY Quality in a Yoga Context

There are many different ways to explore this. The tips below are a starting point for your exploration; this is not meant to be an authoritative or exhaustive text! I hope you'll feel free to develop your own approach, use of the tools, and understanding.

When

When I see or experience the following, I want to increase the heavy guṇa:

- Season: fall, windy days
- Behaviours: agitation, anxiety, overwhelm, not sleeping through the night (or at all)
- Use this guṇa for grounding, anchoring, building, and nourishment

Pace

Try slowing the pace of the class. Moving slowly gives students more time to feel their own weight and its dance with gravity. When the pace is too fast, it feels lighter (the opposite of heavy) and sometimes spinny if we are moving at a faster pace where we lose stability.

Language and Approach

The heavy quality creates a sense of grounding. By using language and cues, you can focus students' attention on feeling heavy, on connecting to the ground and the earth. Experiment with deepening your voice a touch too, letting the tone drop a bit.

When you're cueing, focus on the parts of the body that are "connected to" the earth, using phrases such as:

- "Sink into the earth."
- "Soles of the feet into the mat."
- "Plug your sitting bones into your cushion."
- "Tummy to the floor."
- "Points of contact with the floor."
- "Rooting into the earth."
- "Let gravity draw you downward."

Using this language helps direct the students' focus downward, and *prāṇa* (vital essence of air—vital life energy) follows focus. A big part of Yoga is developing concentration so that we know how to focus our *prāṇa* well and encourage it to move the way we want it to. When our focus is down and our *prāṇa* moves downward (*apāna vāyu*), we feel a sense of grounding.

Another approach is to cue a pose from the top down and leave students' attention at the floor, to give an experience of *prāṇa* moving downward through the body to the floor (*prāṇa* follows focus). Try inviting students to feel the pull of gravity and how that gives them a sense of heaviness and grounding. When cultivating the heavy quality in *Tāḍāsana* (Mountain), cue downward:

- "Feel your feet sinking into the earth."
- "Allow your muscles to soften so you can feel your bones being drawn heavily down by gravity."

- "Stack your leg bones under the bowl of your pelvis."
- "Feel your shoulder blades sliding down your back."

Āsana (postures)

Focus on the bones of the body. Talk about the skeleton instead of the muscles in each *āsana* you teach. It's not about the *āsana*—it's about what the *āsana* allows the teacher to convey and the student to experience. *Āsana* is simply a vehicle for the teachings. So you can use these ideas, teaching any pose from *Sukhāsana* (Easy) to *Parivṛtta Svarga Dvijāsana* (Revolved Bird of Paradise).

The bones are the deepest tissue, and when our bones are healthy, and we allow them to navigate well with gravity, they move downward. They feel heavy. Try including more standing poses and legwork. Getting the legs to work moves our *prāṇa* downward and toward the floor.

Focus on the bowl of the pelvis, where the *mūladhara* (root energy) resides. The pelvis is the foundation of the spine, the root of all spinal movements. By spending time focused on the pelvis, you can cultivate a sense of safety, which leads to stability, which allows students to ground—all connected to the heavy quality. From the pelvis, you can incorporate the legs[19] to continue moving the energy downward and feel into the weight of the legs.

To support students in feeling grounded, cultivating heaviness, use a downward *dṛṣṭi* (gaze or focal point):

- the floor

19 The femurs are the biggest and *heaviest* bones of the body.

- seam between the floor and the wall
- front edge of your mat
- depending on the pose, one's foot or big toe

With a downward focal point, our *prāṇa* moves down toward the floor.

It really isn't about the pose. You can choose any pose. It's how you teach the pose that emphasizes a particular guṇa.

Prāṇāyāma (breath work)

In terms of *prāṇāyāma*, work with the same principle of grounding to cultivate the heavy guṇa. There are some breathing techniques that flow the energy downward very effectively. My favourite is Diaphragmatic Breathing—it's my go-to. It's a very grounding breath if you focus on moving the *prāṇa* into the bowl of the pelvis (root energies). When I'm trying to cultivate more of the heavy quality, I work more with Diaphragmatic Breathing than with the Three-Part Breath because in the Three-Part Breath the energy moves up more. See how choosing a guṇa to emphasize almost picks the techniques for you?

You can use other techniques as well and alter the pacing to cultivate more heaviness instead of lightness. An example is *Kapālabhāti* (Shining Skull Breath). It is a more "lightening" breath. However, if you slow down the pace, it feels heavier and more grounding.

Dhyāna (meditation)

Years ago, I studied iRest Yoga Nidrā with Richard Miller. One of the techniques he uses, which I had not picked up on until I took Āyurveda training, is to invite people to connect with the pairs of opposites in meditation. You're asked to notice where in your body you're feeling light then notice where in your body you're feeling heavy. To increase the heavy quality, allow your attention to rest in the area that feels heavy.

As a result, I teach a basic Yoga Nidrā meditation in every class. If there's a particular quality I'm trying to cultivate, I'll make sure to include that pair of opposites in the meditation then people can compare and contrast their own experience of those particular guṇas. Then I invite them to focus on a particular one and allow their attention to rest there. You can experiment with this in your classes.

Another option would be a *Mūlādhāra Cakra* (Root Cakra) meditation, or any form of meditation that focuses on the sensation of the body's connection to the earth (sensing meditation, walking meditation). You could also do meditation with the eyes open to maintain connection with the earth element through the eyes, using a downward gaze.

Mantra (sacred sound)

Given that *mantra* are seeds of potential energy and manifestation, there is an innate power and potency to this practice. Generally speaking, all *mantras* are *guru* (heavy) with knowledge and potential.

Repetition of the *mantra* gives more weight in terms of knowledge of the *mantra*. As for specific *mantras*:

- The *Guru Mantra* and *Wahe Guru* have the word *guru* in them.
- *Bīja Mantra* (Seed Sound) for the earth element "laṃ."
- *Om* is considered to have all the *mantras* within it, making it heavy.

Mudrās (gestures)

Joseph LePage wrote a wonderful book on *mudrās*, which you can find in the references section. You can use this resource, or your Google search engine, to get more details on each *mudrā*.

In terms of *mudrās*, there are a few *mudrās* that are very grounding. Generally speaking, *mudrās* where the palms are facing downward emphasize grounding.

The first one that comes to mind is *Bhu Mudrā*[20] (Base Element Gesture).

Another *mudrā* I adore for cultivating my connection to the earth element that embodies the heavy quality is *Pṛthivī Mudrā* (Earth).

Integration of the Practice

For the postures of integration themselves, experiment with offering a choice of poses that have more of the body connecting to the earth. This helps to cultivate that sense of

20 Based in the root of the Sanskrit word *bhūta*, meaning the elements.

connection and heaviness. *Śavāsana* (Corpse) with soles of the feet on the wall for additional grounding works well.

You can invite students to use heavy blankets, sandbags, and beanbags to allow them to feel some heaviness in the body during this part of the practice. Lengthen the integration so students can move slowly and deeply embody the qualities that come with this part of the practice.

While students are in their posture of integration, invite them to notice the parts of their bodies that are in contact with the earth and sink into those points of contact, to let gravity make them heavy and surrender to that pull.

If you do a body scan or guided relaxation, move from the head to the feet to ground the energy, or from the upward-facing part of the body (sternum) down through the body (heart and lungs) and toward the floor (upper back).

B. LIGHT GUṆA

If we go to the opposite end of the continuum, we work with the **LIGHT** quality.

Environment / Nature

In nature, the light quality is related to the fire, air, and ether elements. This means not only does lightness manifest as part of weight, but due to its connection to the fire element, also as sunshine and brightness.

The dictionary defines *light* in two broad categories—one with respect to sight (illumination) and the other with respect to weight. In terms of weight, which is what Āyurveda is describing, *light* means: "of little weight; easy to lift" and "requiring little mental effort; not profound or serious."[21]

We find lightness in sand, rainbows, flowers, birds, feathers, paper, hummingbirds, and flies.

In the weather, lightness manifests as sunshine, wind, fluffy snow,[22] sprinkling rain, and in fast-moving clouds.

Body

In the body, this guṇa manifests as a light or a thin frame or a slim build. In the realm of too much or excess lightness of the bone tissue, we see osteopenia and osteoporosis, referred to

21 "Light," Google, accessed March 2018, https://www.google.ca/search?q=Dictionary.

22 Big difference from wet snow!

in the medical community as "light bones." Emaciation is a sign of excess light guṇa. We might also see fair or shiny skin or bright eyes. The Āyurvedic texts describe bright-light intolerance as an expression of excess light guṇa.

Those who have a lot of lightness tend to have challenges with sleep because they don't have enough of the heavy quality to settle in and sleep through the night. So we might notice lightness through scanty sleep or bouts of insomnia.

Mind and Emotions

A sense of lightness in the *mind* allows us to be alert and attentive. Too much lightness in the mind creates a feeling of being spacey, ungrounded, unstable, insecure, fearful, or anxious.

Cultivating the LIGHT Quality in a Yoga Context

When

When I see or experience the following, I want to increase the light guṇa:

- Season: snowy winters, spring
- Behaviours: sluggish, lethargic, depressed, can't get out of bed
- Use this guṇa when you sense that they are "carrying a heavy load" in life, or you want to focus on *en"light"enment* (expanded states of conscious awareness)—a goal of Yoga

Pace

Teach at a faster pace to get things moving. This increases the sense of lightness through speed and movement.

Language and Approach

One approach to creating more lightness in class is the use of humour, keeping things light. I'm a Laughter Yoga teacher and a very cheesy, sarcastic person, so cultivating the light quality this way works for me. It's something I need to be mindful of when cultivating the heavy quality (less humour). Humour can lighten the mood, the energy, and the flow. I use a louder voice with a slightly higher pitch.

Āsana (postures)

Teach the *āsanas* in a way that lifts upward. An example is the version of *Tāḍāsana* (Mountain) where the focus moves from the floor up to the crown and includes cues such as:

- Lift your toes.
- Feel the arch of your feet lift upward.
- Draw the energy from the earth up your legs into the bowl of your pelvis.
- From a neutral pelvis, feel your spine lengthen upward.
- Lift the sternum upward.
- Feel the top back crown of your head float skyward.

With all this upward movement, *prāṇa* follows focus, and when the *prāṇa* moves upward (*udāna vāyu*), we naturally feel lighter. This will work for any pose.

The way I explored lightness this week with Warrior 3 was to start students in *Uttānāsana* (Standing Forward Fold):

- Connect to a sense of lightness in your torso to ***lift*** it parallel with the floor.
- From here ***float*** the back leg upward.
- Feel the lightness in your body, the space in your torso as you elongate your crown away from your back heel.

I also use more arm movements within the poses to create more flow and a sense of connecting to space, which is light in quality.

The focal points move upward to the walls, ceiling, and sky.[23]

Prāṇāyāma (breath work)

In terms of breath work, *prāṇāyāma* tends to be lightening by its very nature. You can use a specific *prāṇāyāma* or choose to cue a *prāṇāyāma* a certain way.

There are specific *prāṇāyāmas* that are lightening in their effect—it is their purpose. For example, *Kapālabhāti* (Shining Skull Breath) and *Bhastrikā Prāṇāyāma* (Bellows Breath or Breath of Fire) are designed to move the *prāṇa* upward and outward. They burn toxins, which literally lightens us internally. These techniques create more clarity in the channels, and this creates a felt sense of lightness. Thoracic breathing (breathing into the chest) is another way of moving energy upward and creating space and lightness in the upper body.

23 Especially if you're teaching outside!

Nāḍī Śodhana (Alternate Nostril Breath) has different effects depending on how you do it. It is typically harmonizing, where you feel an overall sense of balance. Yet you can use Alternate Nostril Breath as a grounding breath or as a lightening breath. The effect it gives depends on things like which nostril you start with, whether you start with an inhale or an exhale, how you use retention, if you use retention, etc. Each of these options has an effect in terms of how the *prāṇa* circulates through the system.

Nāḍī Śodhana is fascinating because you can use it to cultivate any guṇa if you know how it works (i.e., to understand the subtle anatomy and *pranic* flows). I love that. Since it is a layer breath, it also depends which breath you are layering it on top of. If the base breath is the Three-Part Breath or *Kapālabhāti*, then *Nāḍī Śodhana* will have a lighter feel to it. If you layer *Nāḍī Śodhana* on Abdominal Breath, you are cultivating the heavy guṇa.

Dhyāna (meditation)

For meditation, as I described for the heavy quality, I work with Yoga Nidrā and introduce this specific pair of opposites. In the case of lightness, "Where in your body do you feel heavy? Where in your body do you feel light? Allow your attention to rest in the area that feels light."

Meditations that focus on the heart (connected to the air element) or the throat (connected to the ether element), including *Kīrtan*, *Mantra Japa* (Repetition of *Mantra*), *Metta* Meditation (loving kindness), or any form of breath-centric meditation. All of these cultivate lightness in the heart-mind.

Mantra (sacred sound)

Mantras you can explore to cultivate more lightness include:

- *Bīja Mantras* for the corresponding elements: "yaṃ" (air) and "haṃ" (ether)
- *Om* as it clears the channels of the mind
- Purifying (clearing) *Mantras* like *Gāyatrī*

Mudrās (gestures)

Any *mudrā* where the palms are opening upward lets us feel the air and ether elements and the lightness of these elements. This includes *Jñāna* (Wisdom), Open Palms, and *Maṇḍala* (Circle) *Mudrā*.

The air element is connected to the Heart Cakra, so try *mudrās* connected to the Heart Cakra such as *Padma* (Lotus) and *Añjali* (Prayer).

The ether element is connected to the Throat Cakra, so focus on *mudrās* connected to the Throat Cakra such as *Garuda* (Eagle) or *Shankh* (Conch).

Integration of the Practice

Choose postures where there is some form of lift from the earth, yet is still supported, like *Salamba Matsyāsana* (Supported Fish), *Supta Baddha Koṇāsana* (Reclined Bound Angle), and *Viparīta Karaṇī* (Legs up the Wall). Each of these poses has part of the body lifted away from the floor.

For the body scan, move from the feet to the head in order to create an upward movement of *prāṇa*. You might skip cues like “sink into the floor,” which cultivate heaviness, and instead use “soften and relax” or “bring awareness to <area of the body>” without giving a direction to it.

In the body scan, spend more time on the face, which is pointing up and away from the floor. Highlight the areas of the body that are touching the air (like the sternum and the navel, tops of thighs and feet) instead of the floor (like the back of the head, back of the heart, the sacrum, and heels). Move their attention up away from the floor to the part of the body that is the highest, which shifts where the *prāṇa* is circulating (e.g., from the back of the heart, up through the chest to the sternum). Invite students to feel the air touching their skin—such a subtle and light sensation.

Notice the importance of the teacher’s choice of focal points and how we invite students to engage their attention. This makes a difference in the quality of the student’s experience based on which guṇa is cultivated.

CHAPTER 2

INTENSITY: DULL AND SHARP

A. DULL/SLOW GUṆA

Environment / Nature

In nature, the dull or slow quality is related to the water element. Water is heavy, and things that are heavy move more slowly. I find it easier to recognize the slow quality—turtles, snails, and sloths. It is also found in the movement of the tectonic plates (the continental plates) that are moving so slowly we don't even notice. Socks, blankets, Play-Doh, round buttons, and Yoga bolsters are all dull—not in the sense of being boring, but in the sense of not having sharpness to them.

The dictionary defines *dull* as "less intense" and "lacking brightness, vividness, or sheen."[24] It defines *slow* as "not quick or fast" and "lasting or taking a long time."[25]

In the weather, slow manifests as long, never-ending days or a slow-moving storm. Dullness shows up as gloomy, cloudy, and foggy.

I feel like the slow quality needs cultivation in our culture because people are moving too fast. In Vedic speak we refer to this as being "*rajasic*." There is so much speedi-

24 "Dull," Google, accessed March 2018, https://www.google.ca/search?q=Dictionary.

25 "Slow," Google, accessed March 2018, https://www.google.ca/search?q=Dictionary.

ness, movement and rushing around—go, go, go—which has consequences to our nervous system! With this in mind, I work with the slow quality a lot in my teaching practice.

Body

This guṇa manifests as being slow in action for folks who walk, talk, and digest slowly. There is dullness in the voice, skin, or eyes. They tend to have an attitude or a demeanour that is relaxed, calm, and quiet. Silence is attributed to the slow quality.

Mind and Emotions

The mind needs to be able to slow down, to unwind in order to settle into sleep, so this quality is very useful here. Some of us process emotions and thoughts more slowly.[26] Some have more dullness in the mind.

Cultivating the DULL and SLOW Quality in a Yoga Context

When

When I see or experience the following, I want to increase the dull and slow guṇa:

- Season: summer, fall, windy season, busy season
- Behaviours: *rajasic*, overthinking, spinning out, panic

26 I know that I need more time to fully understand, digest, and integrate ideas. I'm not "quick on my feet" that way.

mode, anger, sharp tongue, sarcasm, not settling into sleep

- Use this guṇa to "dull the sharp edges" of anger and panic or to "under-stimulate"/"under-whelm" over-thinking, *rajas*, spinning out

Pace

Teach at a slower pace. Invite the students to move more slowly—nothing fast. Sometimes I start teaching at a regular pace then I slow the pace as the class goes on, so students can feel themselves slowing down. Other times I invite students to do slow shifts and subtle micro-movements in the postures themselves, or a slow flow where it takes a few breaths to move from one pose to the other. Slow transitions from pose to pose. The cue "Roll your spine up in a race to be the *slowest*" is a common way of cultivating more slowness.

I not only slow my cues, I stretch them out and leave a lot of pauses (space) between the cues. The slow quality is connected to quiet. Having a quieter class cultivates dull/slow: more quiet moments in the class, more meditation, and more time for the integration.

An important aspect here is that there is no rush—no rushing at all in any way—through the entire practice.

Another way to explore dullness is to move your attention to an area you can't feel or notice as much and let your attention rest there.

Language and Approach

Experiment with teaching in a monotone voice with less fluctuation and more consistency.

Perhaps dullness is cultivated over time through repetition: doing the same thing over and over as a way of underwhelming the mind and senses.

Emphasize grounding and the downward focus because heaviness slows us down. You will likely notice that the qualities are connected. Here is another guṇa connection—heavy and slow/dull.

Āsana (postures)

I find all the postures fascinating; none of them are "dull" to me in the boring sense. By working with postures that are simple and basic, though, you can avoid activating or over-stimulating the mind: *Tāḍāsana* (Mountain), *Vṛkṣāsana* (Tree), *Daṇḍāsana* (Staff), *Baddha Koṇāsana* (Bound Angle), *Sukhāsana* (Easy Pose), Constructive Rest Pose (not classical, no Sanskrit; it is a physiotherapy option), *Makarāsana* (Crocodile), and *Śavāsana* (Corpse).

Prāṇāyāma (breath work)

Breath awareness is a great exercise for slowing down by anchoring attention to one thing instead of many. I also appreciate Diaphragmatic Breath because it is simple, grounding, and calming. Invite the students to take as long as they need to for a full breath in, take as long as they need to for a full breath out, and any pauses in between.

You can work with any breath and slow it down. Explore a really slow *Kapālabhāti*, where instead of 60 "pumps" per minute, you do 20. A student was telling me about a class where they did timing for *Kapālabhāti* breaths, starting at four counts per in and out breath then changing the pace. To cultivate slowness, you could start at two counts per in or out breath then slow it down to four counts per. As we slow the techniques this way, we can really feel the inhales and the exhales.

Dhyāna (meditation)

Meditation, in most of its forms, is a great way to slow things down.

If I'm working with Yoga Nidrā, I will include this pair of opposites. Dullness is often embodied as an area with less awareness, less feeling, or decreased sensation. Slowness can be felt in bodily processes like heart rate and respiratory rate.

For other meditation techniques, I would go with something that has a more diffuse focal point. Perhaps it would be holding your entire body in your awareness (global awareness) instead of a specific place (like the nostrils).

Mantra (sacred sound)

Repeating the *mantra* slowly cultivates the dull/slow guṇa. Also, since the dull quality is connected with the water element, try water's *Bīja Mantra* "vaṃ."

Mudrās (gestures)

Choose any *mudrā* that resonates, given the context of class, and take your time to talk students through it, reminding them there's nowhere else to go and there's nothing else to do. All they need to do is be present in their practice.

Go with something simple that involves the whole hand instead of specific fingers, like palms to thighs or *Añjali* (Prayer).

Integration of the Practice

I believe the integration of the practice very much cultivates the quiet, slow, dull qualities. Take more time for integration. Invite very slow, mindful, and deliberate movements. Don't use bells or chimes, as they can be sharp. Leave more time for silence.

Many restorative or supported poses work well here, like *Sālamba Śavāsana* (Supported Corpse), *Sālamba Supta Baddha Koṇāsana* (Supported Reclined Bound Angle), or *Viparīta Karaṇī* (Legs up the Wall). Use bolsters and blankets to add softness, which dulls the senses.

B. SHARP/PENETRATING GUṆA

If we go to the opposite end of the continuum, we work with the **SHARP and PENETRATING** quality. An object's ability to penetrate is a result of its sharp quality.

Environment / Nature

In nature, the sharp and penetrating quality is related to the fire element.

The dictionary defines *sharp* as "having an edge or point that is able to cut or pierce something" and "sudden and marked" and "precisely."[27] *Penetrating* is "able to make a way through or into something" and "succeed in understanding or gaining insight into."[28]

We find sharpness in a lion's roar, the peaks of mountains, sharp turns on roads, swords, knives, and teeth. I also think of those sounds that cut right through you, penetrating to the depths of your being. This one is different for everyone—maybe it's fingernails on a chalkboard, or a child throwing a tantrum.

In the weather, sharpness manifests as brisk wind, quick change in weather patterns (was sunny and bright then quickly it is dark and stormy), lightning and thunder, or

---

27 "Sharp," Google, accessed March 2018, https://www.google.ca/search?q=Dictionary.

28 "Penetrating," Google, accessed March 2018, https://www.google.ca/search?q=Dictionary.

freezing rain.[29] It also shows up as the warm sun penetrating your skin, or the damp penetrating your bones.

Body

Physical features can have these qualities. Think of a tapering chin, sharp teeth, distinct eyes, a pointed nose, or a heart-shaped face. Sharpness in the digestion leads to strong hunger. Where the digestion is too sharp (excessive), ulcers happen.

Mind and Emotions

Emotionally, sharpness is anger, rage, resentment, shame, and guilt.[30]

In the mind, sharpness manifests as a strong memory, and strength in terms of understanding, comprehension, concentration, and learning. Think of avid students who have a strong hunger for knowledge, experience, and life—they go deep into the material (penetrating). When taken to the extreme, this attempt to feed the fire of the mind, beyond the body's ability to sustain it, leads to burnout.

This is another quality that is strongly connected to Yoga. When considering Patañjali's *Aṣṭāṅga Yoga* (eight limbs of practice), the eighth limb is *samādhi*, which translates to "absorption." This absorption refers to sustaining your meditative focus long

29 Especially when the bits of ice hit your face!

30 Sometimes guilt can feel dull too. I suspect that it depends on the person.

enough to *penetrate* the object of meditation—to understand it at a deeper level.

Cultivating the SHARP and PENETRATING Quality in a Yoga Context

When

When I see or experience the following, I want to increase the sharp and penetrating guṇa:

- Season: spring, heavy winter, gloomy, cloudy, foggy, long-lasting rain and clouds
- Behaviours: not listening (cut through the mental blocks/obstructions), lethargy, heavy, dense, thick, foggy, bored/dull, hard time getting out of bed in the morning
- Use this guṇa to "cut through" the *tamas*, illusion, habits, dullness, obstructions, distractions
- Caution: be careful to practice *ahiṃsā* when using the sharp and penetrating guṇas.

Pace

Use a faster pace to create a more warming practice, as the sharp and penetrating qualities are related to the hot guṇa.

Language and Approach

Try being less invitational (e.g., "When you are ready, step back") and more directional (e.g., "Step your right foot back"). Strongly hold the container of the space through your presence, focus, and awareness, constantly observing, connecting, and offering feedback.

I generally tend to approach teaching as an opportunity to educate[31] the students, and this is really important when cultivating the sharp quality. Folks who embody this quality want to learn, understand, and know. They want more from a class than a bunch of poses lumped together—they want to dive deeper into the practices, theory, understanding, and experience. They are interested in the method (penetrating).

Being seen and acknowledged offers the student an opportunity to feel the presence and connection to the teacher, which is another way to convey the penetrating quality.

Precision in cueing is paramount in cultivating the sharp quality, where each cue supports the blade of discernment in the mind, cutting away the fluff and flourish. I use very matter-of-fact language, and we get right down to business. I speak more sharply[32] so that the inflection of every cue really lands, which allows the information to penetrate.

I might use more Sanskrit to get their minds working a little more, in response to different sounds and words.

31 I'm not leading them through a practice; I am teaching them Yoga tools.

32 While still being loving and caring—*ahiṃsā*!

Āsana (postures)

I teach the *āsanas* in a very precise anatomical way, describing which movement is happening at which joint and in which order. When cueing *Tāḍāsana* (Mountain), I would use the following cues:

- The bowl of your pelvis is in a neutral position. No tucking the tail under, and no sway in the low back.
- Femurs neutral, no external and no internal rotation.
- The midline of the thigh bones point forward.
- Ground your weight through your heels.
- Spread the weight through the toes—equal amount of weight in the ball mounds of the big toe, baby toe, right-side heel, left-side heel.
- Your spine stacks while maintaining its natural curve.
- Bring your chin parallel to the floor.
- Shoulder blades relax down the back, away from the ears.
- Extend through the tips of the fingers down toward the floor.

I don't cue pose names, but the movements required to get us into and out of the poses.

Choose more complex postures that require the focus and attention of the mind, like *Parivṛtta Trikoṇāsana* (Revolved Triangle), *Svarga Dvijāsana* (Bird of Paradise), *Garuḍāsana* (Eagle), and *Naṭarājāsana* (King Dancer).

I also create a flow of three to five poses and teach the flow then have students move through the flow on their own to engage their mental fire while I walk through the room and assist. I also choose the lesser-known flows (like Moon Salutations instead of Sun Salutations), or I blend flows (Sun Sal R + Moon Sal R, then Sun Sal L + Moon Sal L) to add challenge and engage their attention—to refine the focus of the mind (no autopilot).

Use poses that are more angular because there is an inherent sharpness in the geometry, like *Trikoṇāsana* (Triangle), *Vīrabhadrāsana* (Warriors), *Baddha Koṇāsana* (Bound Angle), *Pārśvakoṇāsana* (Side Angle), and *Koṇāsana* (Wide Angle). There are many different ways we can apply the concept of sharp and penetrating.

Asymmetrical balance poses are great to cultivate the sharp and penetrating qualities—mostly sharpness because one leg is doing one thing, and the other leg is doing something different. One arm is over here, and the other arm over there. Asymmetrical postures require that students pay more attention, and this cultivates mental acuity (sharpness).

Another interesting approach for sharp and penetrating is to work with compression poses where you feel that compression deep inside, like *Bālāsana* (Child), *Kapotāsana* (Pigeon), *Anjayenāsana* (Lunges), and *Mālāsana* (Squat). These poses penetrate the deeper tissues, which moves the focus deeper inside.

Instruct eyes open, not closed, and focused on specific places. The *Aṣṭāṅga* practice is amazing this way with its *dṛṣṭis*—tips of thumbs or nose, looking right or left.

Prāṇāyāma (breath work)

Continue with precision and focused attention. Use breath counting—inhaling to the count of four and exhaling to the count of four.

This is an ideal time to use the more intense *prāṇāyāmas* like *Bhastrikā* and *Kapālabhāti*. Be clear in your instructions, as well as with cautions. It's important to remember that although our language is directional, not all techniques are appropriate for all students. Have a suitable alternative for folks who may be harmed by an unsuitable technique.

We could also blend *prāṇāyāma* with *āsana*, increasing complexity and the need for focused attention. An example is *Deviāsana* (Goddess) with the arms in goal post position and using the *Simha Prāṇāyāma* (Lion's Breath*)* simultaneously—sound, angles, focus.

Dhyāna (meditation)

Use a meditation technique that is contained and precise. The one I like to use is called *Shamata*, which means "calm abiding" in Tibetan. My Buddhist meditation teacher, Larry, taught this technique. From your meditation seat, the focus is to count the exhalations from 1 to 10 and then 10 to 1 over and over. It creates a really strong container. It allows you to notice your ability to stay focused. The first time I counted to 14, I was like, "Oops!" I lost my focus; I lost the sharp quality in my mind. It is a different type of container than "Watch your breath." How do you know when you've drifted off and for how long? See the difference in sharpness?

Use meditations that are connected to the *Maṇipūra Cakra* (Navel Cakra) or the fire element. An example of this is *Tonglen* Meditation, where we take in the suffering of the world and use the fire of our hearts to transform this energy into something that we want to give back to the world. Also explore *trāṭaka* (candle gazing), which is accessible to students of all levels of practice.

Mantra (sacred sound)

A more penetrating practice is a more disciplined practice, something like a 40 or 100-day practice of a *mālā* (garland or string of counting beads, which refers to 108 repetitions).

To connect to the energy of the fire element, one could chant:

- the *Bīja Mantra* "raṃ"
- any of the "Rama" Mantras

Mudrās (gestures)

Think angular and more complex. The complexity might be in the *mudrā* itself, like *Gaṇeśa Mudrā* (Gesture of the Elephant). Perhaps it's a *mudrā* where the hands are holding different shapes/patterns. Doing *mudrās* behind the back, like reverse *Namaste* (Prayer), requires us to pay more attention because we cannot see our hands and what they are doing.

Integration of the Practice

For integration, I focus more on the penetrating aspect of this quality. How can I get students to go deeper inside, to connect to themselves and the wisdom that exists within?

From *Sālamba Matsyāsana* (Supported Fish) or *Supta Baddha Koṇāsana* (Reclined Bound Angle) or *Viparīta Karaṇī* (Legs Up the Wall)—still angles and not quite as soft and supported as *Śavāsana* (Corpse)—as I guide students into integration, I connect them to their heartfelt desire, to their inner teacher that has the wisdom. Perhaps I leave them with a question so they can self-inquire, or they ask their own question from their inner teacher. It keeps them focused and present—instead of being "tuned out," they are "tuned in."

CHAPTER 3

TEMPERATURE: COLD AND HOT

When I work with students, cold and hot are the qualities I start with. Everyone gets the idea of hot and cold and has had experiences of these qualities. This exploration is what started me down the path of Guṇa Yoga.

A. COLD GUṆA

Environment / Nature

In nature, the cold quality is related to the water and air elements.

Cold is defined as "of or at a low or relatively low temperature, especially when compared with the human body" and "lacking affection or warmth of feeling; unemotional."[33]

The cold quality is found in ice, sub-zero temperatures, raw foods, and dairy products.

In the weather, cold manifests when the temperature is below zero[34] and in ice, snow, freezing rain, and fall and winter seasons. There are also cool breezes, which are a sweet relief in the summer.

33 "Cold," Google, accessed March 2018, https://www.google.ca/search?q=Dictionary.

34 I live in Canada, where zero degrees Celsius is freezing!

Body

If we embody the cold quality, we are likely to have cold hands or feet, muscle stiffness, and clammy skin. Our digestion slows down too. Numbness comes from too much cold quality, which is why people put ice on their body to numb that area. Too much cold quality impairs the circulation and flow of fluid and heat in the body. Catching a cold is too much cold quality.

Mind and Emotions

Coldness manifests as insensitivity.[35] Unconsciousness, which is a lack of presence or strong numbness, is cold. Fear and insecurity are also connected to the cold quality.

Cultivating the COLD Quality in a Yoga Context

When

When I see or experience the following, I want to increase the cold guṇa:

- Season: summer, warm climates and temperatures
- Behaviours: irritation, frustration, anger, rage, *rajas*, overheating, hot flashes, and night sweats
- Use this guṇa to "cool off" and "cool down"

Pace

Use a pace that does not build heat in the body. One approach to this is to slow things down.

35 As in the expression: "That person is very cold."

Language and Approach

I approach the practice with thoughts of "easy does it" and "cool, calm, and collected." I give the students more breaks and resting poses.

I focus on using and cueing the bones to support the poses, as opposed to engaging muscles. When we use the muscles, we build heat in the body.

Āsana (postures)

There are areas where heat naturally releases from the body, specifically the armpits, groin, and mouth. Incorporate *āsanas* that allow this movement of heat out of the body.

Using the groin as an example, incorporate wide-legged and straight-legged poses into the practice. The wide legs allow the heat to release from the groin. Straight legs use less muscle energy, which reduces heat. This includes poses like *Prasārita Pādottānāsana* (Wide-Legged Forward Fold), *Utthita Tāḍāsana* (Five-Pointed Star), *Trikoṇāsana* (Triangle), and *Baddha Koṇāsana*[36] (Bound Angle).

Another place where the heat likes to vent is the armpits, hence why we end up with sweat marks under the arms in the summer and at the gym. To cool the body down, we use goal post arms, arms above the head, arms out to the sides, or arms forward—anything that creates some space under the armpits so the heat can release and the body cools down.

Incorporate more forward folds, as forward folds are more

36 The knees are bent, but the legs aren't weight bearing, so the quads are relaxed.

cooling to the body and mind. Postures like *Prasārita Pādottānāsana* (Wide-Legged Forward Fold), *Upaviṣṭa Koṇāsana* (Seated Wide Angle), *Prasārita Bālāsana* (Wide-Legged Child), and *Pārśvottānāsana* (Pyramid).

In terms of inversions, *Sarvāṅgāsana* (Shoulderstand) and *Halāsana* (Plow) are considered cooling, as well as *Viparīta Karaṇī* (Legs Up the Wall).

Prāṇāyāma (breath work)

The simplest cooling breaths are the Sighing Breath and *Simha Prāṇāyāma* (Lion's Breath). Heat escapes through the open mouth, and the tongue gets cooled off, which feels really nice. I also teach the cooling breaths—either *Śītalī* (Cooling Breath) or *Śītakarī* (Hissing Cooling Breath).

An important piece to remember when trying to cool down is to make sure you're breathing fully, yet in a gentle and non-aggressive way. For example, using *Dirgha Prāṇāyāma* (Three-Part Breath, or Two-Part Breath if the three parts isn't available) to air out the lungs and torso for the heat to be moved out. We want to ventilate and aerate the body throughout the whole practice.

Dhyāna (meditation)

The use of cooling visualizations can increase the cool quality. This includes walking outside at dawn before the sun comes up, or a walking under the stars at midnight, or moon bathing, which is very cooling and calming to the system.

You can use Yoga Nidrā to have people tune into an area of their body where they feel cool.

I often use sensing meditation, specifically the feel of the flow of the air in the nostrils. The in-breath is cooler than the out-breath, so I have students focus on the temperature of the air as it is inhaled into the body.

Mantra (sacred sound)

The following *mantras* cultivate the cold guṇa:

- *Bīja* Mantra "aim"
- Any of the *Soma* or Lunar *Mantras*, like "Om Eem Shreem Somaya Namaha"
- Element *Bījas*: "yaṃ" (air), "vaṃ" (water)

Mudrās (gestures)

Use *mudrās* where the fingers are spread and the palms are open to let the hands air out, and feel the air on the skin.

Integration of the Practice

Generally speaking, the integration portion of the practice is cooling, as students are less active. Offer *āsanas* that are supported, cooling, and wide-legged. Examples include a Wide-Legged and Wide-Armed *Śavāsana* (Corpse, where the arms and legs come right off the mat), *Salamba Supta Baddha Koṇāsana* (Supported Reclined Bound Angle Pose), *Prasārita Viparīta Koṇāsana* (Wide Legged Legs Up the Wall, use a strap around the femurs to keep the legs from opening too wide).

Make sure the forehead is slightly higher than the chin, which cools the forebrain. The use of eye bags is cooling for the eyes (darkness is cooling). Turn the lights down, if it's an option. For a cooling class, I don't offer heavy blankets, as they are warming.

B. HOT GUṆA

If we go to the opposite end of the continuum, we work with the **HOT** quality.

Environment / Nature

In nature, the hot quality is related to the fire element.

Hot is defined as "having a high degree of heat or a high temperature."[37]

We find heat in fire, the desert, hot springs, friction, ovens, irons, cooked foods, spicy foods, and warm drinks.

In the weather, heat manifests as heat waves, warm winds, sunshine, and summertime.

Body

The most obvious is a warm body temperature—some people just run hot or are referred to as "warm blooded." Gray hair and baldness are considered signs of heat in the head area that burns the colour out of the hair or burns the roots of the hair and the hair falls out, respectively. So where people are gray or balding, that's seen as excess heat. It also manifests as a strong appetite, digestive fire, absorption, and circulation.

---

37 "Hot," Google, accessed March 2018, https://www.google.ca/search?q=Dictionary.

Mind and Emotions

When there's an excess of heat, people become irritated, angry, impatient, and enraged. They might also express passion.

Cultivating the HOT Quality in a Yoga Context

When

When I see or experience the following, I want to increase the hot guṇa:

- Season: fall, winter
- Behaviours: lonely, disconnected, depressed, frigid
- Use this guṇa to "warm them up" and to "warm up to them"

Pace

To build heat, I teach at a faster pace. The more we move, the warmer the body gets.[38]

Language and Approach

The practice has more movement—movements that engage the muscles. I use "rhythm and repetition" to increase heat. A great example is a *Vinyāsa* practice.

I also make sure there is ample *Pratapana* (Stoking the Fire = warm-ups) for the body, breath, and mind. The practice builds, so it doesn't feel like we are on fire; instead, we are gradually

38 The mind too—they are connected!

building heat in a sustainable and manageable way. Building heat in a non-sustainable way depletes the body-mind, which is a chronic issue in North American culture. Sometimes we use healing tools in a way that makes us sick.

Āsana (postures)

Allowing the legs and arms to be wide cultivates a cooling effect, so I teach poses where the feet are together and the inner thighs are together to keep the heat in. Examples include *Tāḍāsana* (Mountain), *Utthita Tāḍāsana* (Palm Tree), *Utkaṭāsana* (Chair), *Paśchimottānāsana* (Seated Forward Fold), and *Bālāsana* (Child—with the inner thighs together).

The same is true for postures where the arms are by the side or the hands are together. An example is *Añjali Mudrā* (Prayer) with elbows hugged into the rib cage.

We do the postures in a way that engages the muscles, like *Vīrabhadrāsana* (Warrior) and balancing poses like *Garuḍāsana* (Eagle) and *Paripūrṇa Nāvāsana* (Boat).

Simple flows, that can be repeated over and over, build heat in the body. One of my favourite simple flows goes like this:

- Start in *Tāḍāsana* (Mountain).
- Inhale up onto your tippy toes into *Utthita Tāḍāsana* (Palm Tree Pose).
- Exhale, lower your heels, bend your knees, and sit back into *Utkaṭāsana* (Chair).

Even the coldest person, if they work with *Utkaṭāsana* long enough, gets warm. My favourite part is when someone stops to remove their zip up because they are too warm to keep it on. Bingo! Repetition of even the simplest flow can create heat in the body.

Another approach is to hold the same *āsana* for a long time—this creates a different heat. If you hold any *Vīrabhadrāsana* (Warrior) long enough, you'll warm up.

Using postures with bent legs, and therefore using more muscle energy, also builds more heat than straight-legged poses. Choose *Utthita Pārśvottānāsana* (Side Angle) over *Trikoṇāsana* (Triangle).

The warming inversions include *Śīrṣāsana* (Headstand), *Vṛścikāsana* (Scorpion), and *Pīñca Mayūrāsana* (Forearm Balance).

A warming *dṛṣṭi* (focal point) includes the eyes open and strong focus to build more *tapas* (discipline).

Prāṇāyāma (breath work)

There are *prāṇāyāmas* that are inherently heating, like *Ujjāyī* (Victorious Breath), *Bhastrikā* (Breath of Fire), and *Kapālabhāti* (Shining Skull Breath).

Some breathing techniques can be modified to become warming or cooling, like *Nāḍī Śodhana* (Alternate Nostril Breath). The left nostril is associated with *iḍā* (lunar channel), and the right nostril is associated with *piṅgalā* (solar channel). Starting the breath with the solar channel cultivates warmth. Layering the *Ujjāyī* on top of *Nāḍī Śodhana* is even more warming.

Dhyāna (meditation)

For visualizations, envision and connect to the sun, a warm beach, or a hot summer day. Using *Metta* Meditation (loving kindness) works to soften and warm the heart. *Maṇipūra Cakra* (Navel Cakra) Meditations enkindle the fire of the belly, which is warming.

Mantra (sacred sound)

Using *mantra* to cultivate *tapas* (the heat of disciplined practice) builds heat within us. A great example is a 40- or 100-day *Japa* (Repetition) *Mantra* practice. You can explore the following *mantras*:

- Heartwarming *mantras* like "Ahim Prema," "Lokah Samastha Sukhino Bhavantu," and "Om Mani Padme Hum"
- Purifying like the *Gāyatrī Mantra*
- *Bīja Mantra* for the fire element "raṃ"

Mudrās (gestures)

Choose *mudrās* that connect to the fire element, like *Sūrya Mudrā* (Sun), and *mudrās* that have closed fingers and palms to retain warmth, like *Muṣti Mudrā* (Fist).

Integration of the Practice

For integration, focus on "warm and cozy." Use heavy blankets for cocooning and making sure the room is warm enough.

Use *āsanas* that keep the legs and arms in, like Constructive Rest Pose and *Śavāsana*, and palms resting on the belly for more containment.

CHAPTER 4
EMOLLIENCE: OILY AND DRY
A. OILY GUṆA

Environment / Nature

The oily quality is associated with the water element. The dictionary defines *oily* as "containing oil."[39] It is found a lot in nature—many plants, nuts, and seeds contain oil, which we extract in order to consume. Examples include essential oils[40] and cooking oils that come from avocado, grapeseed, coconut, sesame, almond, olive, etc. We also find oil in machinery, as it serves a lubricating function. My family owns a garage, and the amount of oil it takes to turn everyone's car into "a finely oiled machine" is wild!

A description of *oily weather*[41] includes "Slightly warm, slightly greasy-feeling, damp. When you walk outside, your skin gets that slimy feeling." I think of it as connected to spring—moist and heavy.

Body

The oily quality is seen in the skin, hair, and feces. Another manifestation is well-lubricated joints. This means joints that don't snap, crackle, and pop. The "Rice Krispies" in the joints

39 "Oily," Google, accessed March 2018, https://www.google.ca/search?q=Dictionary.

40 Often coming from plants like lavender, tea tree, basil, cedar, etc.

41 My bestie, V, described oily weather this way.

are actually an indication of dryness in the body, which is the opposite quality to oily. Those with oily as a quality will have ample moisture in their bodies and have a smoothness about them—in body and even in demeanour.

Mind and Emotions

The oily quality is connected to relaxation, compassion, and love. I find this a sweet manifestation of a guṇa.

Cultivating the OILY Quality in a Yoga Context

When

When I see or experience the following, I want to increase the oily guṇa:

- Season: late summer, fall, dry winter
- Behaviours: lonely, disconnected, non-responsiveness, not as invested, lack of integration of body-mind
- Use this guṇa for cohesion, integration, nurturing, and loving connection

Pace

With an understanding that compassion and love are oily, pace the practice in a way that allows time for nurturing and self-love. In my experience, this would be a slower-than-average pace, and a consistent pace. Emphasizing *ahiṃsā* (non-harming) removes any pushing, forcing, or over-efforting.[42] If we approach the practice from a really loving place,[43] we are cultivating oiliness.

There is a fine line between juicing up our joints and using up our resources. To increase the oily quality, we want to lubricate without overdoing—the building of *ojas* and the using of *ojas* is a unique balance found from person to person. As soon as we overdo, we are using up our *ojas* instead of building it.

Language and Approach

Ahiṃsā is "love, reverence and compassion for all beings,"[44] which perfectly embodies the oily guṇa. Use a language and approach that emphasize *ahiṃsā*, compassion, love, self-care, and nurturing.

Another way to look at oily is "juicy." With a strong emphasis on lubrication to cultivate oiliness, I think of increasing oily as "getting juicy." My students resonate with this language, and most of them want to feel juiciness in their bodies. In this context, you could also consider: What is a juicy and engaging topic/format/theme for the students you work with? And how do we use the Yoga tools to support a connection to this? This could also be a way to build oiliness or juiciness for them.

Practicing in community, a group class, or with friends—sharing the experience with loved ones—is another way to make the practice more oily, juicy, and loving.

42 Although I'm not clear how any of those things are Yoga in the first place.

43 Think *ahiṃsā*.

44 Nischala Devi, *The Secret Power of Yoga* (New York: Three Rivers Press, 2007).

Āsana (postures)

As someone who embodies a ton of the dry guṇa, I work with the oily guṇa a lot. I do this by moving the body in a way that secretes synovial fluid into the joint cavities, which means a good amount of *pratapana* (warm-ups). I use simple warm-up type flows throughout the entire practice.

An example is *Sūrya Namaskārāsana* (Sun Salutations). For some students, Sun Salutations are a warm-up, while other students need a warm-up before doing Sun Salutes. When I am focused on increasing the oily quality using Sun Salutations, I repeat the transitions three or four times each. The flow looks like this:

1. *Tāḍāsana* (Mountain).
2. 4 *Sūrya Prāṇāyāma* (Sun Breaths—inhale arms up, and exhale arms down).
3. Inhale into *Utthita Tāḍāsana* (Extended Mountain), and exhale into *Uttānāsana* (Standing Forward Fold).
4. Inhale into *Ardha Uttānāsana* (Halfway Lift), and exhale into *Uttānāsana*. Repeat four times.
5. Inhale R foot back into *Anjayenāsana* (Lunge), and exhale stabilize *Anjayenāsana*.
6. Inhale extend the front L leg into *Pārśvottānāsana* (Pyramid), and exhale bend the front L knee until it lands over the ankle in *Anjayenāsana*. Repeat four times.
7. Inhale step the L foot back into *Caturaṅga Daṇḍāsana* (Plank), and exhale into Table Top.

8. Inhale into *Go* (Cow), and exhale into *Durgā* (Cat). Repeat four times.
9. Inhale into *Go*, and exhale into *Adho Mukha Śvānāsana* (Downward Facing Dog). Repeat four times.
10. Inhale R foot forward into *Anjayenāsana*, exhale stabilize *Anjayenāsana*.
11. Inhale extend the front R leg into *Pārśvottānāsana*, exhale bend the front R knee until it lands over the ankle in *Anjayenāsana*. Repeat four times.
12. Inhale step the L foot forward into *Uttānāsana*, exhale soften forward.
13. Inhale into *Ardha Uttānāsana*, and exhale into *Uttānāsana*. Repeat four times.
14. Inhale, and exhale roll the spine up to *Tāḍāsana*.
15. 4 *Sūrya Prāṇāyāma* (Sun Breaths—inhale arms up, and exhale arms down).
16. *Tāḍāsana* (Mountain).

Doing a Sun Salutation (or Moon Salutation or Earth Salutation) in this way invites a lot of juiciness into the whole body. It creates smoothness between the movements and the breath. It creates the space for self-compassion by flowing within each part at one's own pace.

The entire practice could have a more relaxing feel or emphasis. You can include a pause for relaxation between each of the poses.

Prāṇāyāma (breath work)

In terms of breath work, I cultivate the oily guṇa by inviting students to smooth out their breath. I do this in any technique that I use—I emphasize a smoothness and a fluidity to the breath.

I always think about pouring out olive oil into a pan and how it flows everywhere. We can create this effect with our *prāṇa*, through *prāṇāyāma*.

I tend toward more relaxing *prāṇāyāmas*, since relaxation is connected to oily, like Diaphragmatic Breathing, *Nāḍī Śodhana* (Alternate Nostril Breath), and *Bhramarī* (Bumble Bee Breath).

Dhyāna (meditation)

Metta Meditation (loving kindness) is a great fit for cultivating love and compassion for the self and others. All of the heart-based meditations are a beautiful choice.

Kīrtan is a good fit for this guṇa. There is a fluidity to it, and as we join our voices and hearts together to chant, it creates a group oiliness, a group compassion, a group connection. Using *Bhakti* techniques, like *Kīrtan*, is all about cultivating love.

Try using Yoga Nidrā to help students tune into an area of their body where they feel oily and juicy.

Mantra (sacred sound)

As you chant, be smooth, slick, and fluid. This is when I let my inner opera singer out. Since the oily guṇa is connected with the water element, explore the *Bīja Mantra* "vaṃ."

Mudrās (gestures)

The heart-centric *mudrās*, cultivating compassion and love, are a good fit here, including *Padma* (Lotus), *Añjali* (Prayer), and *Hṛdaya* (Heart Centre).

Also, choose *mudrās* that help students relax. One student may feel relaxation gets cultivated through familiarity (relaxing into what they know). For another, it could happen through grounding *mudrās* like *Bhu* (Base Element), *Cin* (Awareness), or *Maṇḍala* (Circle).

Integration of the Practice

Many *āsana* practices have one relaxation at the end, and if this is the case, make it loving, compassionate, and juicy.

Another way of exploring this is to integrate more than one integration/relaxation opportunity throughout the practice. In Sivananda and Bikram Yoga, students take "mini-integrations/ *Śavāsana*" as the practice unfolds.

B. DRY GUṆA

If we go to the opposite end of the continuum, we work with the **DRY** quality.

Environment / Nature

In nature, the dry quality is related to the air element.

Dry is defined as "free from moisture or liquid; not wet or moist."[45] We see dryness in deserts, sand and sandpaper, crackers, and cereals (flakes, puffs, etc.). Some grains like millet and buckwheat are drying, and even green veggies have a drying effect in the body, causing constipation. Many cleanses and cleansing foods are drying to the body.

In the weather, there are dry seasons when all the moisture disappears (dries up). Here in Ontario, Canada, we see dryness in the fall for sure, then sometimes in the summer (can be hot and dry), and sometimes in the winter (very cold and dry). The latter two are variable, since sometimes our summers are warm and moist; the same is true with winter. Where there is heat, there is evaporation, which results in dryness.

Body

Dryness shows in the body in our skin, hair, lips, and tongue—we feel the dryness as the moisture disappears. It is present in

---

45 "Dry," Google, accessed March 2018, https://www.google.ca/search?q=Dictionary.

a hoarse voice and coughing. Dryness also manifests as dehydration, constipation, and pain in the body.

Mind and Emotions

In the emotions and mind, dryness is connected to fear, nervousness, anxiety, and especially loneliness. I also see it in a "dry" sense of humour.

Cultivating the DRY Quality in a Yoga Context

When

When I see or experience the following, I want to increase the dry guṇa:

- Season: spring, rainy, humid or moist weather
- Behaviours: cloggy, soggy, unhealthy attachments, depression
- Use this guṇa to dry up clogs, obstructions, and attachment

Pace

Faster movements emphasize the air element, which is drying. Explore teaching a faster-paced practice.

Language and Approach

I cue in a direct and precise way—no fluff and no muss or mush. I use my dry sense of humour—if it's part of who you are, might as well use it.

To dry out the body, I teach a more challenging practice—whether it is more challenging in terms of the poses (increase the complexity), the sequence, or the number of repetitions (e.g., instead of two Sun Salutations, doing five).

Hot Yoga is very drying, given the amount of sweating and moisture loss. This is a great practice for increasing the dry quality.

Since loneliness is a manifestation of the dry quality, practicing alone cultivates dryness, while practicing in community cultivates oiliness/juiciness.

Āsana (postures)

Use *āsana* to cultivate dryness by challenging the practitioner: teach a new *āsana*, use an unfamiliar way of teaching a familiar *āsana*, hold an *āsana* for a long time,[46] or create a sequence with less fluid/smooth transitions. A practice with less fluid transition could go from seated to standing, prone, supine, standing, crouching, seated, prone. Most teachers over time group all the poses from one category together,[47] which creates a smoothness and fluidity to the practice. Choosing not to do this creates a "rougher" practice, one that is more dry.

Prāṇāyāma (breath work)

Generally speaking, *prāṇāyāma* is drying, as all breath work is working the air element. Particularly the fiery breaths,

46 If we're sweating, the body is losing moisture.

47 All the standing poses in one section, all the seated poses in one section, etc.

especially when done with vigor, are very drying and challenging, like *Kapālabhāti* (Shining Skull Breath), *Bhastrikā* (Bellows Breath), or *Ujjāyī* (Victorious Breath).

From the Āyurvedic view, the *Kumbhaka* (Breath Retention) after the inhalation is nourishing, and the retention after the exhalation is cleansing or drying.

Dhyāna (meditation)

For visualizations, feel the warm sand beneath you, a warm breeze around you, or imagine yourself in the desert.

Use the "oily and dry" qualities in Yoga Nidrā.

Practicing a meditation technique that is strict and firm, like Zazen, is a good choice here.

Mantra (sacred sound)

Try the *Bīja Mantra* for the air element, "yaṃ."

Mudrās (gestures)

Explore *mudrās* that connect to the air element, like *Prāṇa* (vital life force) or *Jñāna* (Wisdom) *Mudrā.*

Integration of the Practice

The integration is plain, simple, and short. Focus on "feeling the air on the skin" to connect with the air element.

CHAPTER 5

TEXTURE: SMOOTH AND ROUGH

A. SMOOTH GUṆA

Environment / Nature

The smooth quality is related to the water element. The dictionary defines *smooth* as "having an even and regular surface or consistency; free from perceptible projections, lumps, or indentations" and "without harshness or bitterness."[48]

In life, sometimes things are smooth and flow with ease, and other times they are rough. I think everyone has realized this contrast at some point in his or her life. Along these lines, I also think of "smooth transitions" as being seamless, calm, and straightforward.

We see and experience this guṇa in smooth peanut butter, the surface of a rock eroded by the water, flat surfaces (a smooth road, trail, and ride), and slippery surfaces like an ice rink.

In terms of the weather, we have smooth sailing, calm waters, and calm skies. My friend V describes it as "one of those days where the clouds in the sky are smooth and the air is not too warm and not too cold. The air is humid, but not unpleasantly so."

---

48 "Smooth," Google, accessed March 2018, https://www.google.ca/search?q=Dictionary.

Body

The manifestations are present in the skin (including lips!), hair, nails, organs, and joints too. Those who have a lot of smooth quality are flexible because they move smoothly from one direction to the next. They transition with ease, so changes in direction are smooth. Those who don't have smoothness, who embody roughness instead, will find it hard to move in a lot of different directions and in a lot of different ways—transitions will challenge them.

Mind and Emotions

Flexibility can also be a quality of a smooth mind too—flexible in thoughts and ideas and beliefs. We'll also see a calm nature and gentle mind in those who are smooth.

Cultivating the SMOOTH Quality in a Yoga Context

When

When I see or experience the following, I want to increase the smooth guṇa:

- Season: fall, ALL season changes (transitional times)
- Behaviours: clumsiness, trauma, "rough day"
- Use this guṇa to "smooth out a rough day or rough time"

Pace

To create a smooth effect, maintain a consistent pace throughout the practice.

Language and Approach

Smooth out the tone and volume of your voice, again using consistency to create a smoothing effect. Try using a softer voice and more invitational tone in your cueing. I find that smooth and soft go together; they are collaborative guṇas.

The approach is a seamless flow, one into the other, so there aren't any distinct breaks from one part of the practice to the other. Each part of the class structure moves easily into the next, whether it's one pose to the next or one aspect or portion of the practice to the next (centering into warm-ups into main *āsana* into relaxation into meditation into final *Om*). It feels like a cohesive whole where it is hard to break out any of the separate pieces.

This is a great time to cue movement instead of pose names—and maybe we don't even stay in a pose longer than a breath before we transition with ease into the next movement.

Āsana (postures)

Given that flexibility is part of smoothness, it makes sense to do practices that cultivate physical and mental flexibility.

For physical flexibility, practice postures that invite more opening to the body, or do a posture in a way that surrenders more to gravity, like forward folds, passive backbends, and twists.

For mental flexibility, explore a new pose, or do the same pose you've always done but in a different way. Here are a few examples:

- Enter into Triangle by coming up from the floor instead of from standing and tilting downward.
- Change the breathing in a flow like Cat-Cow: Instead of inhale into the backbend and exhale round your spine, try exhaling into the backbend and inhaling to round your spine.

Doing things differently creates more flexibility, not only in the body but in the mind as well. Creating new grooves in the mind (*saṃskāra*, neuroplasticity) allows us to be more flexible and adaptable.

I once was in a class where we were invited to move "with the grace of a dancer," and it struck me that this invites us to "smooth out" our movements.

Prāṇāyāma (breath work)

This one is as simple as focusing on a smooth breath. Focus on a really smooth in-breath and smooth out-breath, and consistently remind the students throughout the entire practice:

- Allow your breath to feel smooth.
- Cultivate ease in your breath.
- How can you smooth out the breath in this pose/ practice?

The technique itself matters less, although it is easier to breathe smoothly in breaths like Diaphragmatic, 2/3-Part, *Ujjāyī*, *Śītalī* or *Śītakarī*, and *Nāḍī Śodhana* than in *Kapālabhāti*. It creates a unique challenge to use a more jagged breathing pattern, like *Bhastrikā* and *Kapālabhāti*, and cultivate smoothness within the rhythm. So fun!

I remind students to feel a smooth flow of their *prāṇa*, regardless of which *vāyu* we are working on. *Prāṇa* follows focus, so smooth mental flows = smooth flow of *prāṇa*.

Dhyāna (meditation)

The transition into meditation is smooth and seamless—we move to seated and begin to focus on the natural and smooth flow of the breath. The meditation techniques that are breath-centric are a great choice for cultivating smoothness, since there is a rhythm and repetition to the natural flow of the breath.

Using Yoga Nidrā, we can focus on this particular pair of opposites, bringing this concept into awareness.

Mantra (sacred sound)

A *mantra* that is familiar feels smooth as we practice it. In terms of specific *mantras*, you can explore the following:

- The Breath *Mantra* "So Haṃ" is said to smooth out the breath.
- *Bīja Mantra* for the water element, "vaṃ."
- "Om Mani Padme Hum" has a smooth grace to it.

Mudrās (gestures)

For *mudrās*, they would integrate into the flow of the practice. You're in the *mudrā*, and you don't have to talk about it being a *mudrā*; you simply cue the palms together in front of the heart, or the thumb and fingertips connect gently on an exhalation. We know it's a smooth transition and movement when being there makes sense, where your body would have moved there on its own.

Integration of the Practice

Integration flows seamlessly from the practice into the posture of integration. Any of the supported postures allow the body-mind to smooth out and relax, especially *Śavāsana* (Corpse) given that it's the simplest of the integration poses. Also consider which integration pose will support the smooth flow of *prāṇa* given the practice.

B. ROUGH GUṆA

If we go to the opposite end of the continuum, we work with the **ROUGH** quality.

Environment / Nature

The rough quality is related to the air element. It is defined as "having an uneven or irregular surface; not smooth or level" and "not gentle."[49] We see it in bumps in the road and rocks, the seams of our clothing, materials like corrugated cardboard and corduroy, sand paper, and transitions that are challenging as well as difficult conversations.

In the weather, extreme temperatures (whether hot or cold) and extreme manifestations of weather patterns (water and waves, rain, snow, wind, storms, hail) are rough.

Body

Here we see cracked skin, nails, hands, feet, teeth, hair, cracking joints, and constipation. It manifests similarly to the dry quality, as there is a connection between the dry and rough qualities.

Mind and Emotions

I am aware as I write this section that the qualities are in the "eye of the beholder" or the "experience of the experiencer."

49 "Rough," Google, accessed March 2018, https://www.google.ca/search?q=Dictionary.

For myself, there are some emotions that are "rougher" for me to experience, like shame, grief, and hurt. I know other people who find anger is what challenges them. We're all different in our perception of what is rough; this is true for every quality.

Rough in the mind for me is "the straw that breaks the camel's back," that point of "I just can't do this anymore," or "I just cannot handle one more challenge." At time, I also notice that my thoughts don't always flow in a smooth and coherent way—they are jagged and all over the place. It's like the container of my mind gets rough.

Cultivating the ROUGH Quality in a Yoga Context

When

When I see or experience the following, I want to increase the rough guṇa:

- Season: spring, wet winter
- Behaviours: *tamasic*—for example, stuck in unhealthy patterns/behaviours, needs shaking up or disrupting of the current state of mind
- Use this guṇa to "shake people out of" unhealthy patterns and stuckness, or to help them "shift gears"
- Caution: be careful to practice *ahiṃsā* when using the rough guṇa

Pace

Vary the pace to create a rough effect—faster at one part, then slow down for another then pick it back up again. Like a graph with ups and downs.[50]

Language and Approach

Try using precise and directive language. I refer to *tapas* (heat or friction of disciplined practice) and the importance of this discipline when it's rough and hard. It is often on the day when it feels too "rough" to practice that we need it most.

With rough and dry being connected, I teach a more challenging practice. This might be more challenging in terms of the poses (increase the complexity), the sequence, or the number of repetitions.

Āsana (postures)

Increase the rough quality by challenging the practitioner. Perhaps teach a new *āsana*, use an unfamiliar way of teaching a familiar *āsana*, or challenge through long holds or through more complex transitions.

Prāṇāyāma (breath work)

Kapālabhāti by its very nature is rougher (less smooth) given its emphasis on the exhalation.

You can also work with *Kumbhaka* (Breath Retention) and the challenge of holding the breath in an easeful way. Doing *Nāḍī*

50 Within reason and in a way that will not create injury to the students, of course.

Śodhana with a staggered pattern of inhales, exhales, and retentions is more challenging/rough: IN 4, RT 16, EX 8, RT 32. Granted, we can do this with many different techniques, including abdominal breathing. Taking a basic technique and adding complexity is a great way of increasing the rough quality.

Dhyāna (meditation)

Using the "smooth and rough" qualities in Yoga Nidrā.

An exploration is to intersperse meditation sits throughout an *āsana* practice. Some folks find it rough to "switch gears" from doing (*āsana*) to being (meditation sit), and back again. Including a few of these switches back and forth challenges students and increases the rough quality.

Use techniques with more complexity—use *mantra*, *mudrā*, visualization, and repetition all at the same time. A great example is the Cakra meditations on the Integrative Yoga Therapy cards by Joseph LePage. We are visualizing the *maṇḍala*, using a specific *mudrā* for the hands, and chanting the *Bīja Mantra* a specific number of times.

Mantra (sacred sound)

Since the rough quality is an attribute of the air element, using its *Bīja Mantra* "yaṃ."

Learning a new, longer, or more complex *mantra*, which is challenging or rough, is a good fit for this quality. Examples of longer, more complex *mantras* include:

- *Gaṇeśa Chalisa*
- *Lakśmī's Śṛī Suktam*

Mudrās (gestures)

Focus on *mudrās* that are more complex, like *Gaṇeśa* (Elephant) and *Yoni* (Womb); also, where the hands are holding different *mudrās*, like Green *Tārā*.

Integration of the Practice

For me, a "rough" integration is a short integration.

You could also ask more of the student by giving them a specific focus during the integration. A few examples include:

- Staying present with the flow of the natural breath instead of tuning out.
- Mental *Nāḍī Śodhana*, meaning alternate nostril breath with no hands.
- Following a specific *prāṇic* flow like the Microcosmic Orbit[51] or Blending the Inner Winds.[52]

An aspect of the guṇas that I deeply appreciate is how there is no good and bad. In the beginning of my Yoga teaching, I would not have considered creating a rough practice. At the time I would have found it "unyogic." Now I am grateful to recognize the balancing value of a technique or approach well applied.

---

51 Bernie Clark, *Yinsights* (Vancouver BC, 2007), 392.

52 Sarah Powers, *Insight Yoga DVD* (Pranamaya Inc., 2005).

CHAPTER 6

VISCOSITY: DENSE AND LIQUID

A. DENSE GUṆA

Environment / Nature

The dense quality belongs to the earth element. It is also sometimes referred to as "thick." In scientific terms, *density* refers to "mass per cubic inch."[53] It's not about how heavy something is, although dense things tend to also be heavy, but how thick it is.

We see density and thickness in concrete, large objects (rocks, buildings, mountains), rainforests (thick plant covering), metals (the densest being osmium), and neutron stars.[54] I am also reminded of molasses, honey, and roast beef—thick, dense foods.

In terms of the weather, we have thick fog and clouds, dense smog, and humidity.

Body

The manifestations of dense and thick are seen in the skin, hair, nails, and feces (bowel movements that clog tend to be dense and thick). Think of a person with compact and

---

53 "Dense," Google, accessed March 2018, https://www.google.ca/search?q=Dictionary.

54 "The densest objects in the universe," ESA, updated Oct. 15, 2002, http://www.esa.int/Our_Activities/Space_Science/Integral/The_densest_objects_in_the_Universe.

condensed tissues, and to stereotype (it is useful) I think of football players and rugby players—how dense and thick their biology is. In these body types, we often see a limitation in the range of motion because there is so much dense tissue that the joints find compression quickly. Firm, solid, and strong muscles are dense.

Mind and Emotions

This quality promotes a feeling of groundedness. It can also manifest as thick-headedness, foggy brain/thinking or a lack of space, movement or flexibility in the mind.

Cultivating the DENSE Quality in a Yoga Context

When

When I see or experience the following, I want to increase the dense guṇa:

- Season: fall, precipitation
- Behaviours: spacey, scattered, and "all over the place"
- Use this guṇa to "bring things back together" (cohesion)

Pace

I can feel my density more by moving more slowly, and so I slow down the pace of the class.

A class feels dense when there are many techniques or practices packed into a short period of time.

Language and Approach

A class feels dense when there is a lot of instruction and information given. Since the dense quality connects to strong tissues, I teach a class that builds strength.

Āsana (postures)

For physical strength, practice postures that use the muscles and build strength. Lots of standing poses (Sun Salutations, Warriors, and balance poses), belly-down backbends, planks, and boats.

For mental strength, I teach a series of poses and how to transition from one to the next then I have students go through the flow on their own, using their memory.

Prāṇāyāma (breath work)

Since the dense quality is grounding, try grounding breathing techniques. The Diaphragmatic Breath is one of the most grounding. *Nāḍī Śodhana* also fits in this category.

Ujjāyī thickens[55] the sound and flow of the breath, making it denser and more grounding.

Layering *Ujjāyī* on top of the Diaphragmatic Breath or *Nāḍī Śodhana* would be a great combination for increasing the dense quality—thickened sound of breath, grounding breath work and multiple techniques at once.

55 Thank you for this one, V!

Dhyāna (meditation)

Choose grounding meditation techniques—Root Cakra, earth element, or any technique that allows you to settle.

On option given in Yoga Nidrā is to recline, which can feel grounding and relaxing, allowing us to feel our density. Focus on the "dense and liquid" pair of opposites as well.

Mantra (sacred sound)

Using the earth element's *Bīja Mantra* "laṃ" connects us to the dense quality.

Longer, more complex *mantras* are more dense. Examples include:

- *Gaṇeśa Chalisa*
- *Lakśmī's Śṛī Suktam*

Mudrās (gestures)

Try a *mudrā* connected to the earth element, like *Bhu*. Include grounding *mudrās* like *Jñāna* and *Cin*.

Integration of the Practice

Use integration postures that allow for a sense of relationship with gravity. I like to use *Viparīta Karaṇī* (Legs Up the Wall), where you can feel the femurs[56] sink into the bowl of the pelvis. Also, *Sālamba Supta Baddha Koṇāsana* (Supported Reclined Bound Angle) has compression in the low back (we

---

56 These are the biggest and heaviest bones in the body.

feel the strength and density of the lumbar vertebrae), and we can feel the density of the bolsters supporting us.

If available, blankets, belly bags or sandbags, and eye pillows may be used to increase students' sense of grounding and connection with the sensation of density through the props.

B. LIQUID GUṆA

If we go to the opposite end of the continuum, we work with the **LIQUID** quality.

Environment / Nature

In nature, the liquid quality is related to the water element. The dictionary defines *liquid* as "a substance that flows freely but is of constant volume."[57] From the Āyurvedic perspective, this involves the idea of dilution, which is the change of a dense and thick material to one that is more liquid or diluted. According to the dictionary, *dilution* is defined as "the action of making something weaker in force, content, or value,"[58] reducing concentration, reducing thickness. There is more space between the component pieces.

We see liquid everywhere—water, soda, tea, coffee, rivers, lakes, and oceans.

In the weather, look for water—rain, snow, steam, humidity, and clouds.

Body

The human body is over 75% water, very liquid. We embody liquid in sweat, urine, thirst, salivation, and mucous. Where

57 "Liquid," Google, accessed March 2018, https://www.google.ca/search?q=Dictionary.

58 "Dilution," Google, accessed March 2018, https://www.google.ca/search?q=Dictionary.

there's excess liquid, it can pool or accumulate, which causes a variety of issues like edema and congestion (mucous build-up) in the chest, sinuses, throat, and head.

Mind and Emotions

Emotions are fluid by their very nature in that they arise, exist, and dissolve. With a connection to the water element, we see liquidity in our tears and sorrow.

In the mind, I see both liquid and diluted. The liquid aspect manifests as the flow of thoughts, ideas, inspirations, and the chatter of my ego. The diluted aspect shows up when I can't focus on something, and in the process of integration.[59]

Cultivating the LIQUID Quality in a Yoga Context

When

When I see or experience the following, I want to increase the liquid guṇa:

- Season: fall
- Behaviours: *tamasic*—stuck, obstructed
- Use this guṇa to "zoom out" to dilute where we are stuck in a perspective, or to "create space" for fluidity and flow.

59 Where something that was once separate dissolves and becomes part of my experience and memory, and sometimes even beliefs and understanding.

Pace

You could use a fast or a slow pace—simply stay consistent in the flow. I believe this quality is cultivated more in the approach than the pace.

Language and Approach

Use a consistent volume of voice and consistency in your cueing.[60] Where your language is more directional, you are guiding the flow; where your language in more invitational, you are allowing for free flow through choice.

I think the definition of *liquid* as "a substance that flows freely but is of constant volume" describes *Vinyāsa* beautifully.

Using postures and sequences the students know creates more ease in the flow, while bringing in new elements/ techniques creates more challenge in the flow—both can be useful.

Āsana (postures)

Instead of long holds, choose either short or long *Vinyāsas* for the students to embody—moving from one pose to another, feeling flow and fluidity. For example, I choose three poses and link them together into a flow that repeats over and over. And as we continue through the flow, it becomes more fluid, hopefully so fluid that you can no longer tell one pose from the other. They dilute into each other—the boundaries of one pose dissolve into the other to become one whole flow.

60 Don't leave them hanging!

We can use this concept of dilution in *dṛṣṭi* as well by going from a specific focal point to a soft global gaze.

Prāṇāyāma (breath work)

Experiment with breath awareness, allowing the inhalation to dissolve into the exhalation, to dissolve into the inhalation, and allowing that flow to keep happening. Also pay attention to the point of transition between the inhalation and the exhalation. Or explore and feel the liquid flowing nature of the breath and *prāṇa*.

Dhyāna (meditation)

In meditation, explore a "global awareness" meditation (focus includes the entire body) instead of a focused attention meditation (concentrating on a fixed point). For the global awareness meditation, I invite students to spread their focus using cues like:

- "Hold all of your body in your attention, all at once. From the crown of your head, to the soles of your feet, and including the palms of your hands." Invite them to spread their focus to hold their entire being in their attention, all at the same time.
- "Feel the space around you." You've got space in the front, in the back, on the top, on the bottom, to the right, to the left, and so it dilutes your attention, yet you are still paying attention. It is simply happening in a different way.
- "Notice the sensation in the palms your hands and then allow your attention to spread through your whole hand.

> Keep your attention in your whole hand, and allow it to spread up your whole arm." I have them slowly diffuse their attention over a broader and broader area, even within their own body.

Try using the "dense and liquid" qualities in Yoga Nidrā.

Mantra (sacred sound)

Liquidity is an attribute of the water element, so we can chant its *Bīja Mantra* "vaṃ."

Mudrās (gestures)

Try *mudrās* that are connected to the water element, like *Yoni* (Womb) and *Jala* (Water). Also focus on flowing from one *mudrā* to another, like *Añjali* (Prayer) into *Kapota* (Pigeon) into *Padma* (Lotus).

You could also work with attention in a diluting way, as was described for meditation. In a *mudrā*, say *Garuḍā* (Eagle), first invite your students to feel the connection between the pads of the thumbs. Then invite the attention to spread to all the fingers then dilute the awareness even more to feel the air on the whole of both hands and fingers.

Integration of the Practice

Have the integration portion of the practice flow easily from the remainder of the practice. Use global awareness meditation in the integration instead of fixed focal points. Guide the students through a body scan that moves from one area of the body to another, or even from one *kośa*[61] to another. Bring their awareness to the natural "flow" of their breath.

61 Subtle anatomy term that relates to "sheath" or layer of the human experience.

CHAPTER 7
COMPRESSIBILITY: SOFT AND HARD

A. SOFT GUṆA

Environment / Nature

The soft quality belongs to the water element. I love the dictionary's definition of *soft*: "easy to mold, cut, compress or fold," also "a pleasing quality that involves a subtle effect or contrast rather than a sharp definition."[62]

Softness is found in kitten and bunny fur, cashmere, velvet, feathers, flower petals, marshmallows, pudding, and mud.

In terms of the weather, I found many articles online about how "soft" often translates to "mild" or "calm" when referring to the weather. We also see it in soft snow, soft rainfalls, and soft fluffy clouds.

Body

The soft quality presents in the skin, hair, nails, tissues, and mucous (considered the softest of the body's fluids). One of the classical texts says, "A pleasing look," which I did not understand until reading the dictionary definition around subtle contrasts versus sharp—soft features in the shape of one's face, body, eyes, and being.

---

62 "Soft," Google, accessed March 2018, https://www.google.ca/search?q=Dictionary.

Mind and Emotions

This quality emphasizes forgiveness, love, compassion, kindness, and tenderness. I also consider softness in the mind a form of malleability and flexibility, or in other words, a lack of rigidity and fixed mind.

Cultivating the SOFT Quality in a Yoga Context

When

When I see or experience the following, I want to increase the soft guṇa:

- Season: fall, winter, hard times
- Behaviours: *rajas*, forcefulness, criticism, perfectionism, fixed mind, rigid body
- Use this guṇa when "life is hard" or to "soften sharpness"

Pace

Use a milder pace, and offer a gentler practice to creating softness.

Language and Approach

Try using a softer voice, and more invitational language. When softening the practice, I give my students lots of choices—they can choose between variations, different poses, which *prāṇāyāma* they want to do, and even resting as needed.

Softening, in my interpretation, involves anything that activates the parasympathetic nervous system. This is the part of your nervous system associated with the "rest and digest" functions. It's less about the specifics of the technique and more about an approach that cultivates safety and ease so the nerves can settle, and the body-mind can relax and soften.

I cultivate the soft quality a lot in my teaching practice. My teacher Dr. Claudia Welch often says, "Life is hard and weird, so it's best to make room for this in your life." I have found this to be true. Sometimes life is really hard. I remember last fall in just one class, my students were experiencing the following life circumstances:

- put my mom in a home, found out my daughter has leukemia, and my dog died.
- my sister has been diagnosed with cancer.
- a scathing and embarrassing article was written about me, and I'm losing my job as a result.

Sometimes life is really hard, and when it is, Yoga doesn't have to be hard too. We can cultivate softness in practice to balance things out. I keep practices and sequences shorter, so it is easier to maintain the calming effect on the nervous system.

Āsana (postures)

Try offering simple accessible versions of the poses. Keeping it simple allows the practice to have a softer feel, and the students can surrender more to the poses and the practices. You can still flow, or hold poses. Again, it's the ease-filled and accessible approach over the specific techniques.

I choose a lot of supported poses[63] as a way of allowing

63 Think Restorative Yoga.

students to feel the softness of the blankets and props, and to practice softening into them. If you have enough, maybe use two mats (put one on top of the other) or a mat and a blanket for more softness.

Prāṇāyāma (breath work)

Try focusing on breath awareness, *Nāḍī Śodhana*, *Ujjāyī*, Diaphragmatic, and Sighing Breaths—all forms of *prāṇāyāma* that most students are familiar with and can "lean into" or soften into. There should be no forcing, no straining, no excess effort, only simple and relaxed breathing with an emphasis on ease.

Dhyāna (meditation)

Yoga Nidrā is a wonderful style of meditation for cultivating the soft quality because the student is guided (held) by the teacher's voice for the entire practice. In Yoga Nidrā the student can choose a reclined or supported pose, which can increase their ability to soften into the practice. This approach to meditation often has the added benefit[64] of being relaxing and supportive.

Open Palm Meditation is another approach that works well. Be aware of and soften the palms open. The idea is to stay present in an open and soft, surrendering way.

Breath Awareness Meditation is another beautiful option. Watch the breath, stay present, and allow.

64 Thank you, Josh! Great choice.

Any of the heart-centered or calming meditations, like *Metta* or *Tonglen*, are beautiful choices.

Mantra (sacred sound)

Chanting simple *mantras* using a soft melodic voice cultivates the soft quality. Specific *mantras* that come to mind are:

- Heart Softening *Mantras* like "Om Tare Tuttare Ture So Haṃ/Swaha," "Om Mani Padme Hum," and "Lokah Samastha Sukhino Bhavantu."
- Feminine *Mantras* that connect you with the energies of *Lakśmī*, *Saraswatī*, *Parvatī*, and *Tārā*.
- *Bīja Mantra* for the water element "vaṃ."

Mudrās (gestures)

Focus on simple *mudrās*. I love the idea of "open palms" or *Jñāna* (Wisdom). One of my favourites is *Hṛdaya* (bringing the hands over the heart).

Integration of the Practice

Spend more time in integration—softening, being supported, and letting go.

I love *Viparīta Karaṇī* (Legs Up the Wall), *Sālamba Śavāsana* (Supported Corpse), *Sālamba Supta Baddha Koṇāsana* (Supported Reclined Bound Angle), and *Dradhāsana* (Side Lying, which feels very safe) with ample props, especially blankets. I have quite a few students who feel safest in *Bālāsana* (Child). The invitation is to feel the softness of the blankets and props and to practice softening into them, to relax/let go/surrender to the support and softness, and to the practice itself.

B. HARD GUṆA

If we go to the opposite end of the continuum, we work with the **HARD** quality.

Environment / Nature

In nature, the hard quality is related to the earth element. According to the dictionary, *hard* is defined as "resistant to pressure; not easily broken, bent, or pierced" and "requiring a great deal of endurance or effort."[65]

The hardest naturally occurring substance on earth is the diamond. There are many other hard substances, some natural and some engineered. These include Kevlar, spider's silk, silicon carbide (used to make tanks), bedrock, cobblestone, and sandstone.

In the weather, look for challenging or extreme weather of any type—ice, storms of all types (ice, wind, rain), heat, drought, etc.

Body

This quality manifests as hard muscles, bones, nails, and teeth. It is interesting because I think people move away from hardness, and yet there are some tissues that are healthiest when they are hard—like the bones, nails, and teeth. You might also see calluses on the hands and feet, which come from hard work (in some cases). Hardness is connected with

65 "Hard," Google, accessed March 2018, https://www.google.ca/search?q=Dictionary.

strength, hence why we might see this in the muscle tissue as well.

Mind and Emotions

What is hard in terms of emotions varies from person to person. Which are the emotions that are the most challenging, the hardest for you to be with and process? I observe that grief is hard for most people. This quality is also connected with insensitivity, rigidity, selfishness, and callousness.

I often listen to Pema Chödrön's audiobooks, and she says, "The opposite of a flexible mind would be a rigid [hard] one."[66] Hardness can be fixed, firm, set, and without movement.

Cultivating the HARD Quality in a Yoga Context

When

When I see or experience the following, I want to increase the hard guṇa:

- Season: spring
- Behaviours: need discipline, lack of respect for self or others, break up the *tamas*, to increase humility
- Use this guṇa to build *tapas*, which is the "heat" cultivated through disciplined practice

Pace

Another way to describe a hard practice is to say it is challenging. I alter the pace, so it is not what the students expect.

66 Pema Chödrön, *Getting Unstuck* (Sounds True, 2005).

For my groups this is a faster-paced class. That said, I was in a power class where the teacher went super slowly and gently, and it was really hard for the regular participants because it was not what they expected.

Language and Approach

My language is directional and my tone is firm. I'm not going to yell at anyone; however, I am not invitational or as soft as I can be.

The approach is to challenge the students. Using postures and sequences the students are unfamiliar with will challenge them. I offer fewer variations. The practice is longer and more challenging, physically and mentally, with a shorter integration period at the end.

Āsana (postures)

Experiment with posture flows with longer holds and doing one side for many poses in a row. For example, in a standing series you might hold each pose for 10 breaths, and flow from one to the next:

- *Vīrabhadrāsana 2* (Warrior 2)
- *Viparīta Vīrabhadrāsana* (Reverse Warrior)
- *Utthita Pārśvakoṇāsana* (Side Angle)
- *Ardha Candrāsana* (Half-Moon Balance)
- Poet's Pose --> variation on *Ardha Candrāsana* (could not find a Sanskrit)
- *Utthita Pārśvakoṇāsana* (Side Angle)
- *Viparīta Vīrabhadrāsana* (Reverse Warrior)

- *Vīrabhadrāsana 2* (Warrior 2)
- Repeat the sequence on the other side

Use postures that build muscle strength while working the bones against gravity (and the pull of the muscles) to build strength.

Practice postures and transitions with more complexity for more challenge, like *Parivṛtta Svarga Dvijāsana* (Revolved Bird of Paradise), *Naṭarājāsana* into *Sthiti Dhanurāsana* (King Dancer into Standing Bow), and *Kākāsana* into *Śīrṣāsana* (Crow into Tripod Headstand).

It's important to consider that what is hard for one group or student might not be for another. For one student, Power Yoga might be hard, and for another it might be Yin Yoga that is challenging. The idea is to offer a challenge, to work with *tapas* to help students grow outside of their comfort zone—whatever that looks like.

Prāṇāyāma (breath work)

There are many ways for breath work to be challenging—longer practice and more challenging techniques. If your class tends to be light on *prāṇāyāma*, perhaps your emphasis is typically *āsana*, having the students work with a formal 5 to 10 minutes of *prāṇāyāma* will challenge them.

Introduce a new technique. I introduced *Bhramarī Prāṇāyāma* (Bumble Bee Breath) to a group last week. The technique itself is not challenging, however many of the students were challenged with making noise[67] in a room full of people, and

67 They come from a "good girls are quiet" generation.

so we did *Bhramarī* in all our seated poses to try on a noisy *saṃskāra* (groove of the mind).

Dhyāna (meditation)

Have a formal sit if that's not typically part of the practice; if it is part of the practice, sit for an extra 5 to 10 minutes. Use techniques that require more focus and attention, like *Shamata* (Calm Abiding) or introduce a completely new technique.

Use the hard and soft pair of opposites in Yoga Nidrā.

Mantra (sacred sound)

Explore chanting the earth element's *Bīja Mantra* "laṃ."

Chanting complex *mantras* and using the classical Vedic intonation for chanting cultivates the hard quality. *Mantras* that come to mind include the *Gaṇeśa Chalisa* and *Lakśmī's Śṛī Suktam*—both are very long, and therefore harder to learn.

A neat one to do as a group is *Mantra Japa* (Sacred Sound Repetition). Working in a group this way brings in a lot of other pieces, like pacing as a group and saying the *mantra* out loud in front of other people. And a *mālā's* worth is a good number of repetitions. You could choose a longer *mantra* that requires learning and remembering, like *Mahā Mritunjaya*, *Asato Mā Sad Gamaya*, or *Gāyatrī*.

Mudrās (gestures)

Teach *mudrās* that are complex, new, or asymmetrical.[68]

Integration of the Practice

What comes to me here is "bare bones." No blankets, bolsters, or cushions.[69]. Have students lying on the floor in *Śavāsana* (Corpse) with more quiet space than talking and a shorter amount of time in integration.

68 Where one hand is doing one *mudrā* and the other hand is doing a different *mudrā*.

69 Too soft.

CHAPTER 8

FLUIDITY: STABLE AND MOBILE

I feel like there's an irony to this pair of opposites as it connects to the world of Yoga. People come to Yoga either for healing (stability) or to touch their toes (mobility). And often for both, the whole process of Yoga creates stability, which gives one more freedom (mobility) in their lives. This pair of guṇas has Yoga written all over them, and in many contexts!

A. STABLE GUṆA

Environment / Nature

The stable quality belongs to the earth element. This goes well with the dictionary definition of *stability* as "not likely to give way or overturn; firmly fixed" and "not likely to change or fail; firmly established."[70] Firmly established is what Patañjali refers to in terms of *āsana*. Stability manifests in nature through consistent rhythms and patterns (cycles), mountains, rocks, and earth (solid ground).

In terms of the weather, stability manifests as consistency within a season or seasonal pattern. Here in Canada we would say a warm summer, windy fall, snowy winter, and rainy spring. These are the patterns we expect, and the patterns that make sense for us. Stability in weather

70 "Stable," Google, accessed March 2018, https://www.google.ca/search?q=Dictionary.

happens when a season expresses as expected (e.g., no snow in June!).

Body

Stability is found in solid joints, bones, and body. People who have a lot of stability have few injuries and illnesses.[71] Their high embodiment of stability means their body is very resilient.

Mind and Emotions

It is the ability to sit quietly, to sleep well, and to do nothing. Without enough stability, there can be no healing or change that takes place in the body. Lasting change only happens when there is solid ground on which those changes can take hold. This is why stability is a quality I often try to cultivate for myself and for my students.

I am excited to write about this guṇa because it is a direct link to Patañjali's Yoga Sūtra 2.46 ***sthiram sukham āsanam***. The translation is "*Āsana* (seat) is *sthiram* (stable) and *sukham* (creates sweet space)." I love this because what it basically says is that without the stable guṇa, there is no *āsana*. You cultivate this sense of stability, and this stability provides the foundation for healing change and transformation for your students.

For me, stability of the heart-mind is mental-emotional stability. This feels like fewer mood swings and fewer unpredictable reactions. The Yogic system is designed to cultivate

71 Although they wonder why everybody else is injured and sick.

sattva (harmony and balance in the mind), and I intend to maintain a connection to *sattva* even when my day is a roller coaster. This takes way less energy than riding the swing of the pendulum between *rajas* (agitation of the heart-mind) and *tamas* (dulling or numbing out).

Cultivating the STABLE Quality in a Yoga Context

When

When I see or experience the following, I want to increase the stable guṇa:

- Season: season changes, fall, erratic weather patterns (unexpected and unpredictable)
- Behaviours: emotional fluctuation, mind all over the place, *rajas*, spilly bendy (lack of containership)
- Use this guṇa to "stabilize the container of the self"—any time you see erratic or unstable movements or behaviour. Knowing that ***sthiram sukham āsanam***, there is no Yoga *āsana* practice without working on stability

Pace

Maintain a consistent pace throughout the class—no speeding up or slowing down. Steady.

Language and Approach

Speak with confidence and maintain a balanced and stable tone throughout the class.

In stability-enhancing classes, try cueing alignment from a skeletal perspective, stacking bones and feeling the play of gravity to navigate more stability in the postures.

Presence is an important concept in teaching—period. However, I believe that the level of presence is really important if we're cultivating stability. The Yoga Teacher acts as a container for the practice. To build stability,[72] presence and containership become more important. Through this, students learn to contain themselves and their own transformation and growth. First we hold the container so they can explore change, then they learn to do this for themselves.

Taking a tangent on the previous footnote around *Mūlādhāra Cakra* (Root Cakra): Not only is stability about stability, but for most animals, it is also about safety. A stability-building class needs to factor in what is happening in the autonomic nervous system—sympathetic (activity; fight or flight) versus parasympathetic (rest and digest). Being in fight or flight does not feel stable, nor does it feel safe. Parasympathetic-enhancing techniques are useful for stability, and therefore healing of the body-mind.

One of the elements I really enjoy when working with this quality is to find stability in instability. Here are questions I invite my students to explore within themselves:

- How do you find stability and balance when you are out of balance?
- Can you find the solid ground inside yourself when the world outside of you is swirling with movement?

72 Which is a huge Root Cakra concept.

- How do you become the eye of the storm?

I find this idea quite useful for life.

Āsana (postures)

I know this was just mentioned, however, 2.46 ***sthiram sukham āsanam***. Without the stable guṇa, there is no *āsana*.

I believe we can offer stability-enhancing classes in two ways: We can do postures that are very balanced to feel balanced, or we can do postures where we must find our balance in order to learn how to build and cultivate stability. Both are useful, depending on which other guṇas are present.

When I want to increase my students' awareness of their stability, or lack of it (both are useful) I use balance poses. It's not just about being stable; it's about being able to find stability when you're not stable. We explore balance in a variety of ways—one-legged poses, one hand and one knee, head, hands and forearms, seat. It can be fun and playful to explore finding balance and stability.

This is the type of class where I guide students to check in more frequently:

- From seated: notice if there's more weight in the right sitting bone than in the left sitting bone.
- From standing on two feet: notice if there's more weight in the heels or more weight in the toes. Can you find somewhere in the middle?
- From prone or reclined: notice where the points of

contact are, and which feels most connected to the earth.

All these explorations that we have done in so many Yoga classes are all to build and cultivate awareness of our level of stability.

Stability is inherently grounding, so choose *dṛṣṭi* (focal points) toward the earth. Cue them to sense into whatever areas of the body are touching the floor/mat/cushion. *Apāna Vāyu* (Downward Moving *Prāṇa*) is very stabilizing for the entire system. Actually, any *dṛṣṭi* (focal points) is stabilizing for the mind, so explore using *dṛṣṭi* for each pose.

Prāṇāyāma (breath work)

Any *prāṇāyāma* that calms the nervous system is stabilizing, like Diaphragmatic, *Nāḍī Śodhana* (Alternate Nostril), 2-Part, and *Ujjāyī* (Victorious). A consistent practice of any technique also cultivates the stable guṇa. The techniques with a steady rhythm are also stabilizing, like *Kapālabhāti* (Shining Skull), *Bhastrikā* (Bellows), *Nāḍī Śodhana* (Alternate Nostril), and *Ujjāyī* (Victorious).

The simplest way, in my experience, is to have the students even out (stabilize) their in-breaths and out-breaths in these or other breathing techniques.

Dhyāna (meditation)

Meditation techniques are designed to stabilize and balance the mind. This is true for all Yoga techniques, actually. All of Yoga is designed to bring stability and balance for the body, *prāṇa*, emotions, mind, and spirit. Thus, any form of meditation cultivates mental stability.

Seated or reclined meditation techniques are very stabilizing since the body is stable and supported.

Techniques with more structure provide more of a container for the students, like Yoga Nidrā, *Shamata* (Calm Abiding), and *Mantra Japa* (Sacred Sound Repetition[73]). Any of the *Mūlādhāra Cakra* (Root Cakra) or calming meditations increase the stable guṇa.

Mantra (sacred sound)

One approach to cultivating stability with *mantra* is consistent practice with the same *mantra* for a long time.[74] Stabilizing *mantras* include:

- *Om*—a foundation chant, also very grounding, simple, and quickly familiar.
- The *Guru Mantra* connects us with the lineage of the tradition of Yoga.
- *Mahā Mritunjaya* is the healing mantra, and we talked earlier about how healing requires stability.
- *Bīja Mantra* for the earth element "laṃ."

Mudrās (gestures)

Try simple, grounding, earthy *mudrās*, like *Bhu* (Base Element), *Cin* (Consciousness), *Jñāna* (Wisdom), and *Maṇḍala* (Circle).

---

73 Repetition is very powerful in terms of calming the nervous system and creating stable patterns in the mind.

74 Like months, years, or even a lifetime.

Integration of the Practice

Spend more time in integration, as this part of the practice promotes parasympathetic activation, which is great for stabilizing the biology and the emotions.

Use postures that provide good support, like *Śavāsana* (Corpse), *Dradhāsana* (Side Lying), *Viparīta Karaṇī* (Legs Up the Wall), and *Sālamba Supta Baddha Koṇāsana* (Reclined Supported Bound Angle). I have a few students who use *Bālāsana* (Child) because this is the one pose where they feel safe and stable enough to relax.

Stay present to your students as they integrate. Send them *ahiṃsā* through your eyes, chant *mantra* quietly, or simply watch over them. Your ability to be present, your containership, affects their ability to be present and engage in the practices. Yoga is demanding as a practice—it's changing us. That doesn't always feel safe or stable. Having a teacher that cares enough to stay with you during the process makes a huge difference.

B. MOBILE GUṆA

If we go to the opposite end of the continuum, we work with the **MOBILE** quality.

Environment / Nature

In nature the mobile quality is related to the air element; think of wind. According to the dictionary, *mobile* is defined as "able to move or be moved freely or easily."[75] Other language that infers the mobile guṇa includes *transformation*,[76] *change*, *active*, *variable*, *unstable*, *restless*, and *erratic*.

Mobility is found everywhere: the movement of the planets in our solar system, phases of the moon, growth cycles, wind blowing, tide coming in (and going back out), running, walking, moving, jumping, dancing, evolving, and breathing (inhale into exhale, exhale into inhale).

In the weather, mobility is high during the seasonal changes, when we're switching from one season to another. Another way the mobile quality shows up in the weather is when something is unseasonable, as in when there is a variation in the seasonal norm (e.g., snow in June). And let's not forget hurricanes and tornadoes!

---

75 "Mobile," Google, accessed March 2018, https://www.google.ca/search?q=Dictionary.

76 I am aware here how the two opposite qualities need each other. In order to have lasting change, there has to be enough stability to hold the transformation. How cool is that?

Body

This quality manifests in movement of all sorts. Think of people who talk a lot, and move their hands while talking. When the mobile quality increases significantly, we begin to see instability or erratic movements (instead of smooth and fluid). Hypermobility is instability in the joints, which means dislocations. Other manifestations include tremors, shakiness, seizures, restless eyes,[77] moving eyebrows, and restless leg syndrome. Folks with a lot of mobility are constantly walking, talking, traveling, multitasking. The mobile guṇa is associated with the *rajas mahā* guṇa.[78]

Mind and Emotions

Mobility in the emotional body is experiencing the flow of an emotion as well as a change in the emotions. Mobile minds have dreams, scattered dreams, lots of thoughts, thoughts all over the place, restlessness, insecurity, anxiety, and erratic behaviour. Mental instability includes mood swings, manic depression, and bipolar disorder.

Cultivating the MOBILE Quality in a Yoga Context

When

When I see or experience the following, I want to increase the mobile guṇa:

---

77 A person who cannot make eye contact or focus on one point.

78 The ***mahā* guṇas** are the three main qualities of *prakṛti*. One of these great qualities is *rajas*, the energy of movement and activity.

- Season: long seasons (e.g., long winter), spring
- Behaviours: stuck in a rut, rigid, fixed, stagnant
- Use this guṇa to "get unstuck" or "get moving"

Pace

Mobility is cultivated well in a *Vinyāsa* (flow) style class. Transitions, moving from one pose to the next, increase the mobile quality, which is why *Vinyāsa* is ideal. Having variability in the pacing also increases the mobile quality.

Language and Approach

Experiment with using invitational language to give the students choice, instead of providing one fixed way. The volume and tone of voice can vary from pose to pose or flow to flow.

In my experience, there is a fine line between teaching a class to increase the mobile quality and destabilizing students. There is such a thing as too much mobility, and so we want to increase mobility without it becoming erratic. The traditional practice of Yoga was designed for freedom, and yet lots of people are using Yoga to get high (destabilized) instead. Having experienced erratic classes, I choose to cultivate mobility within a container of consistency and stability.[79] We spend more time and focus on transitions and repeat transitional movements a few times to cultivate an aptitude for safe and conscious transitions. Another way to think of this

79 To me, this feels safer. I am a safety-first teacher. Other teachers will cultivate other things based on their priorities and values.

is increasing flexibility within an appropriate range of motion (ROM)—not so mobile that we create injury.

I use repetition a lot in classes to enhance mobility. I have students flow from one pose to the next; however, the series of poses creates a container for the movement so it doesn't become erratic. An example of a simple flow series is:

- *Vīrabhadrāsana* (Warrior 1)
- *Pārśvottānāsana* (Pyramid)
- *Parivṛtta Trikoṇāsana* (Revolved Triangle)
- *Pārśvottānāsana* (Pyramid)
- Repeat the flow five times on one side then switch sides

Āsana (postures)

Mobility is very much connected to flexibility, and so the practice focuses on flexibility over strength.

Since *Vinyāsa* is ideal, there aren't any long holds in the practice. Instead, there is more movement; there are more postures and more transitions from posture to posture. In each pose, I teach a flow of sorts. An example is:

- Come into *Vīrabhadrāsana* (Warrior 1) legs.
- With each inhalation, the arms flow forward and lift up to the sky.
- With each exhalation, we bow forward from the hips over the front leg, and the arms extend forward and down until they are in line with the torso.

The legs are stable, and the upper body flows. You could add more flow by extending the front leg on the inhalation and sinking back into *Vīrabhadrāsana 1* legs on the exhalation. And within this, I would change the *dṛṣṭi* from inhale to exhale. On the inhalation, the *dṛṣṭi* is at the seam of the wall and ceiling in front of you, and on the exhalation the *dṛṣṭi* is the big toe of your front foot.

Ask yourself: "How much mobility do I want to cultivate?" and "How can I do it while maintaining stability?"[80]

Prāṇāyāma (breath work)

Prāṇāyāma is all about containing and building *prāṇa* then learning how to move it through the body in ways that enhance health and consciousness. Each technique moves the *prāṇa* in different ways. A few examples include:

- *Nāḍī Śodhana* (Alternate Nostril) is an amazing technique for bi-lateral flow and regulating the *vāyus*.
- Abdominal breathing encourages the increase of *apāna vāyu* (downward-moving energy), which is why it is grounding and stabilizing.
- Thoracic breathing increases the flow of *prāṇa vāyu* (*prāṇic* ingestion flow) and *udāna vāyu* (upward-moving *prāṇic* flow), which is energizing.
- *Kapālabhāti* (Shining Skull) is a more vigorous *prāṇāyāma*; therefore, there is more *prāṇic* movement with this technique. This technique emphasizes *udāna vāyu* (upward-moving energy) and *samana vāyu* (centering energy).

80 I refer back to Patañjali's Yoga Sūtras—*sthiram sukham āsanam.*

Dhyāna (meditation)

Since *prāṇa* and mobility go hand in hand, use meditation techniques that focus on the movement of the breath.

I love the 61-point relaxation technique where you are guided from one *marma* (vital energy point) to another in a sequential way, and your attention rests on one point until you are guided to the next point. The focus moves from place to place. However, it is in a precise order, and it uses paced timing.

Another useful option is moving meditation, which includes:

- *Āsana* practice: for *āsana* as a moving meditation, in my experience it is best to give the students a flow they can remember then have them work within the flow.
- Body Sensing: this is where you use simple movements while maintaining strong awareness in one area of the body. You could try a series of Sun Breaths while feeling the sensations in the palms of your hands the whole time. If you lose your ability to feel your palms, then you slow down until you can hold that awareness.
- Walking: For walking meditations creating a circuit to walk works great. I've done this with people going at their own pace (passing happens) and also cultivating a group pace (which is ego-balancing).
- Nature: I love using walks outside as a nature meditation where you consciously look at the blooms in the spring, the changing of the leaves in the fall, the smell of the

warm grass in the summer, and feeling the snowflakes on my cheeks in the winter.[81]

Mantra (sacred sound)

One approach to cultivating mobility with *mantra* is more fluidity and exploration of the sounds, like in *Kīrtan*. *Mantras* you can explore for mobility include:

- The transition mantra "*Asato Mā Sad Gamaya*"
- *Bīja Mantra* for the air element "yaṃ"

Mudrās (gestures)

Create a "*mudrā* flow," where students move from one *mudrā* to another. While in each *mudrā*, take the time to focus on and feel the *prāṇic* flow.

Integration of the Practice

Choose postures that emphasize *prāṇic* flow and fluid breath. The body becomes still; however, the breath and *prāṇa* continue to move. *Supta Baddha Koṇāsana* (Reclined Bound Angle), *Viparīta Karaṇī* (Legs Up the Wall), and *Śavāsana* (Corpse, with shins supported) work well for this.

As part of settling in for integration, try a body scan to move the students' attention in specific ways:

- To raise their *prāṇa* (energy), we scan from the soles of the feet to the crown of the head.
- To ground their *prāṇa*, we scan from their crown to their

81 I'm Canadian, in case anyone forgot or is wondering where to get snow for this experiment. We just have it here.

soles, or from the front of the body toward the back body.

- To circulate their *prāṇa*, we inhale into the heart and exhale the *prāṇa* out to the periphery.

With *prāṇa* being mobile, using *prāṇa* as a focal point during the integration process maintains mobility during stability.

CHAPTER 9
DENSITY: GROSS/OBVIOUS AND SUBTLE

A. GROSS/OBVIOUS/BIG GUṆA

Environment / Nature

The gross quality, also described as big and obvious, relates to the earth element.

The dictionary describes *gross* as "general or large-scale; not fine or detailed" and "very obvious; blatant."[82] *Obvious* is described as "easily perceived or understood; clear, self-evident, or apparent."[83] *Big* is described as "of considerable size, extent, or intensity."[84]

We see this quality in the Rocky Mountains, the Grand Canyon, the Great Barrier Reef, and the trees in Stanley Park in British Columbia.[85] Houses, cars, elephants, whales, and hippos are all things (and beings) that are big in size.

---

82 "Gross," Google, accessed March 2018, https://www.google.ca/search?q=Dictionary.

83 "Obvious," Google, accessed March 2018, https://www.google.ca/search?q=Dictionary.

84 "Big," Google, accessed March 2018, https://www.google.ca/search?q=Dictionary.

85 Google this. The trees are so big that they have dug out space for you to drive your car through the trees!

In terms of the weather, the gross quality shows up in the bigger weather patterns like storms that move across the globe, or a high-rated earthquake. Also, in the obvious—when it's raining, it's raining. If it's warm, it's warm. When it's cold, it's cold.

Body

Grossness manifests as things that are large in size—frame (very tall or stout), bones, hands, feet, nose, and eyes. They are all things that are gross, big, and obvious. Obesity is an excess of the big quality.

Mind and Emotions

This quality means that a person is not able to hide how they feel.[86] People feel how they feel, and it is obvious/written all over them.

They might also feel their emotions more because they are so obvious. Another interpretation is that the emotions might feel "big" to them. This can also manifest a big or very dramatic personality.

Cultivating the GROSS Quality in a Yoga Context

When

When I see or experience the following, I want to increase the gross guṇa:

86 A modern way of saying this is that a person "has no poker face."

- Season: beginning of a season change, when I'm not quite sure what the weather is doing
- Behaviours: "blissed out," spacey
- Use this guṇa to "know what you don't know" and become embodied. One of my favourite ways to work with this guṇa is to consider how to bring the subtleties of Yoga practice into awareness, to make the subtle obvious.

Pace

Maintain a consistent pace throughout so the rhythm of the class is obvious.

Language and Approach

Use simple language and be as clear, concise, and straightforward as possible. One of my favourite quotes is from Albert Einstein: "If you can't explain it to a six-year-old, then you don't understand it yourself."[87] I imagine I'm teaching my nephew[88] or a beginner group. Intend to teach each pose using only three cues to connect with the obvious aspects. Keep the practice simple. Make the intention obvious.

Cue using the obvious structures of the body, using simple language:

- Reach your arms wide.
- Spread your fingers.

---

87 "Quotations from Albert Einstein," Working Minds, accessed Sept. 4, 2018, https://www.working-minds.com/AEquotes.htm.

88 Who is, at the time of writing this book, nine years old.

- Step your left foot back.
- Look over your right shoulder.

When you want to cultivate the obvious quality, use your class time to review the important elements of practice including *yamas*[89] (restraints), *niyamas* (observances), *dhyāna*, and *prāṇāyāma*—not only *āsana*.

Āsana (postures)

Try using poses with obvious names and specific geometric shapes. Invite students to look around to see why the pose is called Triangle or why we call this Head-to-Knee Pose.

I teach the fundamental poses of the practice and remind students why these are the basic foundations for all the other poses. If we explore something more complex, we go back to the basic shape to remind ourselves of the connection to simplicity. I really enjoy Judith Lasater's book *30 Essential Yoga Poses*; it's a great reminder that a lot of practice can happen from 30 basic poses.

Or, if you have a talent for making the complex simple, use it! Take a complicated pose and break it down into simple, doable steps.

89 I think of *ahiṃsā* (non-harming) as the most obvious Yoga practice. However, I am also aware that it is obvious to me, but not necessarily obvious to everyone.

Prāṇāyāma (breath work)

Stick with the basics—Breath Awareness, Diaphragmatic Breathing, and *Ujjāyī* (Victorious). I also like to use Breath Counting to make the breath and its rhythm more obvious.

Dhyāna (meditation)

Rely on basic Seated Breath Awareness Meditation. It is simple and obvious like the pictures on the cover of *Yoga Journal* and the air purifier adverts at Rona.

Mantra (sacred sound)

Chanting out loud, versus whispered or internal practice, is more obvious. Experiment with *Lithika Japa* (Written Repetition of Sacred Sound). Try the *Bīja Mantra* for the earth element "laṃ."

Mudrās (gestures)

Practice simple *mudrās*, like Open Palms, *Jñāna* (Wisdom), and *Maṇḍala* (Circle).

Integration of the Practice

Śavāsana (Corpse) is the classic and most familiar posture of integration. No fuss, no muss. Lie on the floor. Soften and rest. Keep breathing and relax.

B. SUBTLE GUṆA

If we go to the opposite end of the continuum, we work with the **SUBTLE** quality.

Environment / Nature

In nature, the subtle quality is related to the ether element. Depending on the text, sometimes also the air element. These aren't seen with the naked eye, only inferred. According to the dictionary, *subtle* is defined as "so delicate or precise as to be difficult to analyze or describe" and "understated."[90] Another translation for *Sūkṣma* is *minute* as in "extremely small."

The subtle quality is the twinkle in someone's eye, fine threads of a silk blouse, beating of a hummingbird's wings, the details of a feather, and fleas.

In the weather, subtlety is when we're not sure what we're seeing, like a fine mist on the water. Or when we wonder, *Is that rain outside?* It is also micro-climates and small weather patterns (it's raining here but not across the street). The small differences in light at different times of day.[91]

---

90 "Subtle," Google, accessed March 2018, https://www.google.ca/search?q=Dictionary.

91 Thanks for these ideas, Gummo. Awesome!

Body

Subtlety manifests as goose bumps, twitches, and fine tremors.[92] *Prāṇa* is very subtle, as not everyone can see it.

The *kośa* (sheath or layers of being) model, or any of our subtle anatomy maps, is a great example of obvious to subtle. According to a five-*kośa* map:

1. *Annamaya kośa* (physical body) is the most obvious
2. *Prāṇamaya kośa* (layer of *prāṇa*)
3. *Manomaya kośa* (layer of emotions, instincts, and unconscious patterns)
4. *Vijñānamaya kośa* (layer of the intellect, intuitive wisdom, and witness consciousness)
5. *Ānandamaya kośa* (layer of bliss) resides closest to *puruṣa* (soul)

Each layer is subtler than the one before it.

At its essence, Yoga is a science of subtlety. As we refine in our practice, we get more and more subtle with it. It starts with "How do I move my body" to "How should my hands be?" to "Where am I looking?" to "How should I breathe?" to "Where do I focus my mind?" As we deepen the practice, we become more and more refined. We get more and more subtle. There are many layers of this subtlety, as described by the *kośa* model like, "How does my *prāṇa* move in this pose? What emotion does this pose evoke? Can I breathe through those? What is my mind doing in all of this?"

92 When your muscles do that little twitchy thing.

I find there are so many wonderful ways to allow people to explore the subtleties within themselves using Yoga techniques. My friend dallas uses the word *nuance* when exploring subtlety in teaching, which is one of her tools to make Yoga more accessible.

Mind and Emotions

A couple of other mental-emotional manifestations of subtlety can be spaciness, anxiety, and insecurity. I believe there is a connection of subtlety to awareness too—sometimes what we are experiencing is so subtle that it is under our level of awareness. For example, I had no idea how anxious and angry I was (for decades), until it became obvious. Interestingly, I didn't get more angry or anxious, I simply wasn't aware, or we could say that it was not obvious to me that I felt this way.

Cultivating the SUBTLE Quality in a Yoga Context

When

When I see or experience the following, I want to increase the subtle guṇa:

- Season: typical seasonal climate
- Behaviours: when I see students with pain and trauma. Those in physical pain benefit from shifting focus to breath; those in mental and emotional pain (could be trauma, could be something else) benefit from moving out of the mind and back into the body
- Use this guṇa to "dive deeper within" and explore

"different levels of self." Yoga and Āyurveda have many subtle anatomy maps one can use for these explorations.

Pace

Connect with the subtle quality through pacing by changing the pacing a little bit at a time over the course of the class. No big changes; little tiny ones as we go.

The natural flow of a class has subtle changes that are inherent to the practice. We practice postures from standing; in the same class we also do postures in reclined, prone, seated, and crouching positions.

Language and Approach

Try using minimal language so students can be more involved in their own experience than in your voice and cues. This allows the students' inner voice to be more obvious. I want students to connect to and experience their inner wisdom, which is a more subtle and quiet voice inside them.

The approach I enjoy, when working with the subtle quality, is to get people to dive in and notice what the practice is doing—what is the *karma* of the practice? After each pose, I guide the students through a series of self-inquiry questions to feel the "echo" or effect of that pose/practice, and to guide them inward:

- What is the effect on your body?
- On your breath?
- On your emotions?
- On your mind?
- Is your intention changing?

To work with subtlety in the practice, cultivate curiosity and exploration. Think: *What happens if?*

I appreciate Yin Yoga as a subtle experience of practice. This is a practice with a strong focus on energy flow through the meridians (subtle energy channels of Traditional Chinese Medicine).

Āsana (postures)

Choose any pose and get curious. An example is to come into *Tāḍāsana* (Mountain):

- Bring your feet one inch closer together and notice what happens. What do you notice about your body, the pose, your breath, the sensations, your balance, which muscles are engaging, and which muscles are relaxing? Can you do the pose this way and maintain stability and ease?
- Go back to the first pose and now bring your feet one inch wider apart. Now, what's happening?

I invite the students' attention to the deeper tissues inside the body, like their joints (feel your femurs in your hip sockets), or their bones (feel your vertebrae stacking), or the flow of their *prāṇa*. Get more subtle as you go.

Prāṇāyāma (breath work)

Prāṇāyāma is all about working with your *prāṇa*, which is a more subtle awareness than the body. How can you use the techniques to connect with this more subtle flow?

Dr. Claudia Welch has a CD entitled *Prāṇa* containing four

exercises to help you become more connected to and aware of your *prāṇic* flows.

Dhyāna (meditation)

Meditation connects to the more subtle aspects of mind and emotions, so meditations that allow you to notice what is arising for you moment-to-moment work well—like mindfulness and *shamata* techniques.

Mantra (sacred sound)

Mantra by its very nature, being sound and energy based, is subtle. If we whisper or do mental repetition, we are being even more subtle with the practice. Using "haṃ," the *Bīja Mantra* of the ether element, cultivates the subtle quality as well.

Mudrās (gestures)

Feeling the *prāṇic* flows in a *mudrā* is inherently subtle, so focusing on this aspect in any *mudrā* works great.

Integration of the Practice

I invite students to choose the pose that resonates with them (connection to their inner teacher) and then I guide them through the same self-inquiry process as I would with any other *āsana*. With that guidance inward, I leave them deeper inside than the physical body (maybe breath awareness, or observing *sattva/rajas/tamas* or feeling into *ānandamaya kośa*, or feeling the intention they set at the beginning of class) for the process of integration.

This part of the practice, where the effects of the entire

practice are absorbed into the self, is inherently subtle. Consider offering a longer integration to allow students to experience this subtle process more deeply.

CHAPTER 10

ADHESION: CLOUDY AND CLEAR

A. CLOUDY GUṆA

Environment / Nature

The cloudy quality, also described as sticky and slimy, is related to the water element. It reminds me of mud, the mixture of water and earth together.

The dictionary describes *cloudy* as “not transparent or clear” and “covered with or characterized by clouds.”[93] *Sticky* is described as “tending or designed to stick to things on contact”[94] and *slimy* is “covered by or having the feel or consistency of slime.”[95]

We see this quality in clouds and cloudy substances (like coconut water), slugs, fish, okra, the sap of a tree (sticky).

In terms of the weather, look for overcast skies and foggy or cloudy days. Notice if the earth is hard or muddy (mud is sticky). Also, when it’s hot, damp, and muggy.

---

93 “Cloudy,” Google, accessed March 2018, https://www.google.ca/search?q=Dictionary.

94 “Sticky,” Google, accessed March 2018, https://www.google.ca/search?q=Dictionary.

95 “Slimy,” Google, accessed March 2018, https://www.google.ca/search?q=Dictionary.

Body

It manifests in the body as mucous, which is cloudy, sticky, and slimy. Stickiness also refers to compact firm joints. A joint that sticks together well, that has good cohesion, as opposed to a joint that dislocates. This quality promotes good cohesion in the body (sticks together) and manifests in someone who has a solid and firm structure (body).

Mind and Emotions

Cloudiness, in the mind and emotions, is connected to a lack of awareness and lack of clarity,[96] like seeing through rose-coloured glasses.

Those who have a lot of cloudy-sticky-slimy guṇa have great cohesion, including in relationships. Those who have a lot of sticky quality love to hug and become deeply attached in their relationships, even "stuck" on someone, for better or for worse.

Everyone needs enough of the sticky quality to retain memory. Each memory is an imprint that sticks in the mind—no sticky, no memory.

Cultivating the CLOUDY Quality in a Yoga Context

When

When I see or experience the following, I want to increase the cloudy guṇa:

96 Which is the opposite guṇa of cloudy.

- Season: fall
- Behaviours: lack of memory, lack of connection to self or others, inability stay in one's own experience (empath)
- Use this guṇa to support memory, and "bring things together" (unify)

Pace

Find a pace that allows the teaching to "stick" in the students' mind. Too fast, and they miss things; too slow, and they might get distracted and miss things. I believe that Āyurveda is the science of "Goldilocks"—not too hot, not too cold, not too hard, not too soft, not too fast, not too slow ... just right.

Language and Approach

Some individuals have enough clear guṇa that they lose the boundary of themselves; they can feel into the experience of others. People with this trait are often referred to as "empaths." For these yogis, it can be helpful to shift the amount of clarity so they can stay in their own experience and stick to their own stuff. Many empaths are challenged with sensory overload because not only do they have their own stuff to process, but they are also working through the experiences and feelings of those around them. By clouding their field consciously and deliberately, empaths can reduce the amount of data coming in and the overwhelm that results from too much input. There is also a whole conversation here around being able to digest our own experiences and then trying to digest the experiences of others (which is really hard because they aren't ours to digest). However, this will have to be another book.

I typically don't want to increase "cloudiness" in the practice, as this defeats the purpose of Yoga.[97] It is helpful for me to recognize this guṇa in my students so I can work on the opposite to bring them into balance. And I do want to increase the sticky guṇa, to work the mind and improve memory. I use repetition to imprint the teachings in the mind of the student. I might repeat using the exact same words (saying things twice), or I might repeat the same concepts using different words.

In my experience, simple language sticks better, as does humour and making students feel seen and heard. Students remember the funny things that happened in class, or the thing that made them smile, or the connection they felt with their teacher.

I use repetition not only in the language but also in the sequencing and practice itself. If we're working on something new, I create a flow that allows for repeated practice. Or I teach something students already know that I want them to remember so they can practice it at home. I say that a lot in class too: "Remember to practice this at home." When Śṛī Pattabhi Jois said, "Yoga is 99% practice and 1% theory," he was working with the sticky guṇa.

Āsana (postures)

Cultivating the cloudy-sticky-slimy guṇa is less about a pose and definitely more about the approach. Repetition, memory, and simplicity in the cues and postures.

97 A science based in self-realization—seeing oneself, and the world, clearly and accurately.

You can also choose non-*dṛṣṭi* or a diffused (cloudy) gaze in the postures instead of a fixed point.

Prāṇāyāma (breath work)

Generally speaking, *prāṇāyāma* is clarifying for the channels of respiration, as well as the *nāḍīs*. And yet if we want the effects to stick, we need consistent repetition of the practices.

Dhyāna (meditation)

Mantra Japa (Repetition) is a beautiful example of a meditation that cultivates the sticky quality. When you first learn a *mantra*, it is challenging, and we often ask ourselves, "What is going on? What is this *mantra*? Why am I doing this?" If you chant a *mantra* regularly for a long enough period of time, it chants itself to you in the back of your mind while you're doing other things. This is how you know it has stuck.

And as with all the techniques in this section, to cultivate a lasting effect of the benefit, repetition of practice is key to helping things stick in the body-mind.

Mantra (sacred sound)

The approach to chanting that cultivates this quality is *Mantra Japa* (Repetition).

Use the water element's *Bīja Mantra* "vaṃ" to connect with this guṇa.

Mudrās (gestures)

Experiment with *mudrās* that correspond to the water element, like *Jala* (Water) and *Shakti* (Goddess) *mudrās*.

Integration of the Practice

The integration part of the practice is a great place to imprint an affirmation, given how open and receptive we become through the practice. Once folks get settled, have them mentally (quietly, internally) repeat their affirmation to themselves as they integrate.

Another option is to play a *mantra* in the background while students are integrating, which also imprints the *mantra* in their field of awareness.

B. CLEAR GUṆA

If we go to the opposite end of the continuum, we work with the **CLEAR** quality.

Environment / Nature

In nature, the clear quality is related to the air and ether elements—neither of which can be seen with the naked eye, only inferred. According to the dictionary *clear* is defined as "transparent" and "easy to perceive, understand, or interpret."[98]

The clear quality is looking into the ocean and seeing right to the bottom to the coral and the fish. Think also of Saran wrap, glass jars, sheer materials like lace, and eyeglasses.

In the weather, clear is found in a cloudless sky that allows us to see the brightness of the sun, moon, stars, and planets with our naked eyes. Or when the water is so clear that you can see right to the bottom of the lake.

Body

Clarity shows itself in the eyes, skin, tongue, and nasal passages when these are unobstructed—the whites of the eyes are white, the skin is clear of pimples and breakouts, the tongue is not coated with a layer of slimy-sticky *āma* (undigested metabolic waste), and the nasal passages are free

---

98 "Clear," Google, accessed March 2018, https://www.google.ca/search?q=Dictionary.

of mucous. My skin is also clear in the sense of being translucent; you can easily see my blood vessels and connective tissues.[99]

A place we see clear a lot nowadays is through excessive cleansing—everything from anti-bacterial everything to being on a dietary cleanse all the time. I find it helpful to remember that cleansing is important, and yet, so is nourishment[100] if I want my body and mind to have the building blocks they need for health.

Mind and Emotions

The clear guṇa manifests in the mind as immediate understanding (information is clear to a person); however, it can also manifest as forgetfulness. If you don't have enough sticky, you're not going to retain the information. Clear seeing is related to *satya* (reality). Yoga practice, in general, is helping us to disentangle ourselves from the *Kleśas* (mental emotional afflictions), which are veils that keep us from seeing life as it really is.

The clear quality manifests in experiences of loneliness, emptiness, void, and isolation.

It also shows up in the "clairs," which refer to the 6th sense(s) of clairvoyance, clairaudience, clairsentience, and so on.

---

99 I joke with my doctor that I'm not pale, I'm "transparent."

100 Āyurveda's first pillar of health is "Nourishment," not cleansing. The second book I'm writing discusses the three pillars of health.

Cultivating the CLEAR Quality in a Yoga Context

All Yoga practice increases the clear quality because Yoga is a practice of clearing debris from the channels of the body-mind. Doing any Yoga increases the clear guṇa.

When

When I see or experience the following, I want to increase the clear guṇa:

- Season: late winter, spring
- Behaviours: preoccupied, obsessed (stuck)
- Use this guṇa to "clear the way" or "clear the channels"—in the body, heart, and mind

Pace

The clear quality is less about the pace itself and more about being clear about why you're using the pace you're using. The clear quality is connected to intention—why are we doing what we are doing.

Language and Approach

Use language and cues that are clear, precise, and simple.[101] Try not to use any extra or unnecessary words in cueing.

The approach is intentional. I explain why we are doing what we are doing so the intention behind the overall practice, or the individual practices, becomes clear to the student. Unless

101 My teacher Susi often says that "simplicity is a form of genius." I try to remember this at all times.

we share this with our students, how are they supposed to know? I tell my students often that there is "method behind the madness." Nothing in a Yoga practice is random, and everything we do has a purpose. I love sharing what that purpose is.

I have my students set their own personal intention for practice at the beginning of every class. In my experience, this teaches us how to get clear on why we practice and what we want from our practice.

Another approach I use to cultivate the clear quality is functional movement/Yoga therapy. I did a class the other day to help my Āyurvedic Yogis become more aware of their muscular overuse. The complaint was that walking was causing them to get sore, so we did a class to clarify where they are doing more work than they need to get the job done. The movements were simple, and everyone started to notice things like:

- "I'm using my hip flexors to adduct my femurs."
- "I'm using my low back to rotate my femur in my hip socket."
- "I think I'm clenching, and I don't know why."
- "My eyebrows are trying to move my legs."

It was a fabulous class, and everyone came away with more clarity around how they move. It gives them something to pay attention to when they are being active too, which cultivates presence and hopefully reduces compensation, overuse and injury.

Āsana (postures)

Choose any pose and get clear about why we practice it. We don't have to know everything, and yet it makes sense for us to know why we do what we do. For example: "Why did I choose to teach Triangle? We're practicing Triangle Pose because I want you to build strength in your legs, to get that great stretch in your top hip and side waist, and to develop core strength. This is why we are practicing triangle." And once I say it, it becomes clear why we are doing what we're doing. If I don't explain the why, how are the students supposed to know?

I often describe Yoga as a process of purification and refinement. The exact words I use are "Yoga clears the channels of the body-mind, so things flow more freely and with ease." *Āsana* practice helps us to remove *āma* (undigested waste materials) from our body-mind.

Prāṇāyāma (breath work)

Prāṇāyāma is inherently clearing for the channels of respiration, known in Āyurveda as the *prāṇa vaha srotas*, and the *nāḍīs* (subtle energy pathways). Doing any form of *prāṇāyāma* will eventually have this effect.

The following techniques purify the following channels:

- *Nāḍī Śodhana* (literally translates to Channel Purifying Breath) clears *iḍā* and *piṅgalā nāḍīs*, and eventually all the other *nāḍīs* too
- *Kapālabhāti* (Shining Skull Breath) clears the frontal lobes of the brain

- *Bhastrikā* (Bellows Breath) clears the lungs
- *Dirgha* (Long Extended or Three-Part Breath) clears the respiratory channels

These breaths are the most purifying, meaning they achieve a clearing effect quickly.

That said, not everyone needs to clear the guck from their pipes quickly, since that can be very intense, and then we have to digest the extra intensity. Being consistent gives us more benefit than being forceful. As one of my favourite Āyurveda teachers says, "slowly and slowly."[102]

Dhyāna (meditation)

Meditation is the technique we use to clear the channels of the mind, known as the *mano vaha srotas*, from undigested waste materials. It is inherently increasing the clear guṇa. All meditation is supportive in this capacity.

Mantra (sacred sound)

The *mantras* that work with the clear quality include:

- *OM*, clears the space around us and our energy fields, especially when chanted three times in a row
- "Om Gum Ganapatayei Namaha," which we chant to clear obstacles
- Seed sound "aim," which clears the mind
- Seed sound "hrim," which clears the emotions
- So haṃ
- Element *Bījas* of "yaṃ" (air) and "haṃ" (ether)

102 I love you, Dr. Rosy!

Mudrās (gestures)

Mudrās that work with the air and ether elements, like *Prāṇa* (vital life energy), *Akāśa* (space), and *Vāyu* (wind), are a good fit for this guṇa.

Integration of the Practice

At the end of practice, experiment with having students check in to see what effect the practice had on their body, breath, emotions, mind, and heart. Guide them to check back in with their intention, the one they set at the beginning of class, to see if the resonance is still there, or if things have changed.

CHAPTER 11

CONCLUSION TO GUṆA YOGA

Contemplations for the Teacher

In the past when I would pick up a Yoga book to read, I felt I had to learn everything in the book. And although that might be true sometimes, it's not always the case. When you picked up this book, you already knew things. Hopefully you were already teaching Yoga and sharing these teachings with the world in your own way. Before you make the mistake of thinking, *I have so much to learn to teach Āyurvedic Yoga*, first I invite you to contemplate the following questions:

1. What is your current teaching style(s)?

Write a list of what you teach and why you teach it. I believe we teach the things we need to know.[103] If this is true for you, by looking more closely at what you are already doing, you will see that you are already working with the guṇas. I want you to *get clear on which guṇas you are already working with*. I believe part of these teachings is innate—we already have this wisdom inside us. I invite you to consider which guṇas you're already working with and why you work with these guṇas. Are these the guṇas you need to balance in yourself?

---

103 At least this is my *dharma* (purpose).

2. Knowing what you know now about Guṇa Yoga, how can you refine how you work with the Yoga techniques to use them with more purpose and intention?

Notice what comes to you naturally. The next stage of refinement is to do it on purpose. To choose your cues more deliberately and your sequence more specifically, and to choose techniques that give you the effect you are seeking. In the case of Āyurvedic Yoga, this means creating a class that actually increases the guṇa you intend to increase (e.g., create a cooling class that actually cools your students down).

Until I learned about Āyurveda, I practiced and taught Yoga as best as I knew how. With the Āyurvedic layer, many of the why's of the practice began to reveal themselves. As you begin to grasp the basics of Āyurveda, you'll be empowered to explore and understand the practices and techniques of Yoga at another level. You'll find that you evolve and mature in your knowledge of why you do what you do, and when you should do something else instead. There's a richness to this "purposefulness." And teaching with this level of intention is powerful.

3. Can you see the guṇas in your life?

If you don't know where to start "seeing the guṇas," start with the weather. Every day look outside and think about which guṇas you are seeing. Recognize the manifestations of the guṇas so you learn which ones to work with. Refer back to the weather section of each guṇa to get a sense of what to look for.

When you see a guṇa in the weather, that's the guṇa you

practice balancing with your classes that day. Plan your class around the guṇa you are seeing in your environment.

When I first started this exploration, I started with temperature. I looked outside and asked, "Is it hot or cold today?" and I would plan my class around that because it felt doable. Eventually I started to see more, which means I incorporated more into my teaching practice.

Once you get familiar with one guṇa per class then start creating classes that balance two guṇas at a time. Some of the "two guṇa" classes I worked with this year were:

- *Hot and humid*—hot, heavy, cloudy weather. Apply the opposites of *cold, light, and clear.*
- *Cold and heavy*—wet snow. Apply the opposites of *hot and light.*
- *Cold, light, and dry*—windy and cold, fall and early winter with light blowy snow. Apply the opposites of *hot, heavy, and oily.*
- *Cloudy, heavy, and wet*—rainy season. Apply the opposites of *clear, light, and dry.*

Remember, the key is to know why you are doing what you are doing. What is the opposite guṇa to the one you are seeing? (Remember that opposites balance!) Which guṇa is being balanced by which technique? How? Why?

4. Which guṇas are you unfamiliar with?

Likely these are outside your comfort zone. You might not embody these, and you might rarely need to balance them. That said, this is the next step in the process: going outside your comfort zone into the areas that could serve your students because it's more about them and less about you.

This means switching things up—your pace, cues, approach, choices of postures, sequences, and techniques. It's important for us to teach what our students need instead of what we like or what is easy for us.[104] If we're going to grow as teachers, we need to go outside our comfort zone (rough, hard, mobile) to try something new and different.

This section of the book is a culmination of five+ years of teaching exploration and amazing feedback from students and peers. You're not going to be able to memorize this. You need to explore, try, consider, and find your own way through Guṇa Yoga. You likely noticed that some of the chapters had more information and details than others. Guess which guṇas I have more practice balancing? Yep—same. Even for me, this is an ongoing process of exploration. I hope you enjoy the exploration as much as I do. I would love to hear what you discover.

I hope you can see how understanding the guṇas, and how to work with them, sets the stage for Āyurvedic integration into a Yoga practice. Understanding the qualities of nature and how to balance them using Yoga techniques is how Yoga and Āyurveda work together. Once you understand how to do this, and can use Yoga to balance the guṇas, your Yoga becomes effective and profound medicine.

104 Preferences reinforce the ego-personality. To connect to spirit, we need to let that go.

SECTION 2

DOṢA YOGA

INTRODUCTION TO DOṢA

Doṣa is a unique concept found at the core of the Āyurvedic teachings. That said, without an understanding of the guṇas (quality, characteristic, attribute), the doṣas are difficult to grasp, and even more challenging to balance.

The Sanskrit word *doṣa* translates to "fault," "blemish," and "that which vitiates other substances when it is vitiated." The doṣas are the bio-energetic factors in the body that promote health when balanced and promote disease when out of balance. They are often used to refer to the disease or imbalance tendencies we are born with. Āyurveda has a specific language it uses to describe these balanced and imbalanced states of being.

Another way of describing a doṣa is to recognize that each doṣa is a specific grouping of guṇas. Our imbalances come from guṇas increasing to a point that causes discomfort, suffering, and dis-ease. This is why understanding the guṇas is important to understanding the doṣas.

This chapter will help you to understand which guṇas are connected to which doṣas and how these guṇas relate to one another. It will also give you more insight into the depth of the concept of doṣa (guṇas + functions + structures) and why it can be confusing for people to understand. It is also a brilliant tool once we do understand it.

Prakṛti

From the moment of conception, each person has a unique blend of the three doṣas. We refer to this as *prakṛti*—a person's basic constitution and tendencies. *Prakṛti* is like a fingerprint, unique to each person. It is the level of expression of *vāta*, *pitta*, and *kapha* doṣas in an individual. When people talk about their doṣa, they are referring to their *prakṛti*.

According to Āyurveda, one's *prakṛti* dictates the diet and lifestyle regimens appropriate to maintaining health, as well as the nature of potential dis-ease, its prognosis, its prevention, and the most effective treatments.

Vikṛti

I really like how Christina Brown describes the concept of *vikṛti* in her book, *A Year of Ayurveda*:

> Superimposed on our underlying prakriti is the way we lead our lives. Life is a never-ending flow of fluctuating factors. In fact, as we move through life, change is the only thing that doesn't change.... This process called life really keeps us on our toes and although the underlying constitution we were born with doesn't alter, the expressions of it do. Our special mix of the three doṣas changes from minute to minute, day to day, and season to season. The doṣas influence how we eat, drink, sleep, work, play, exercise, and express ourselves. Climate, season, time of day and stage of life all have an effect too. This day to day variance, like a layer superimposed on prakriti, is called vikruti. Vikruti refers to the temporary states of flux in the doshas.[105]

Āyurvedic Yoga is the use of Yoga techniques (*āsana*,

105 Christina Brown, *The Ayurvedic Year* (North Adams: Storey Books, 2002), 15.

prāṇāyāma, *dhyāna*, *mantra*, etc.) to bring *vikṛti* (flux) closer to *prakṛti* (natural balanced state).

Everyone is made up of all five elements, and therefore has all three doṣas to some degree. This is reflected through the sub-doṣas—where various tissues and systems of the body are associated with specific doṣas based on function.

As my teacher Hilary describes:

> By understanding the elements, the doṣas, and the qualities of each, you can begin to negotiate the world around you through direct observation and through application of these simple principles. By cultivating an understanding of how each guṇa affects each doṣa you will begin to open to the simple Āyurvedic practices, which will bring daily balance to your life.

There are two powerful factors that affect the doṣas; these are *environmental changes*[106] and *food*. The good news is we can control our diets[107] and our indoor environments. The outdoor environment is more challenging to change.

The reason we practice Āyurvedic Yoga is to balance the qualities, and therefore the doṣas. When the doṣas are balanced, they convert to their purest forms:

- *vāta* becomes *prāṇa*—the essence of vitality and energy
- *pitta* becomes *tejas*—the essence of brilliance and understanding

106 Like the weather and seasons.

107 In theory …

- *kapha* becomes *ojas*—the essence of immunity and inner strength

An important element to remember is that **every doṣa can practice every pose**. It is *how* we practice the pose that determines the effect, either balancing or deranging for a particular doṣa.

Doṣic Cycles

All the doṣas are active at all times (i.e., each cell in the body is created with a blend of *vāta*, *pitta*, and *kapha*), so it is a matter of degrees of activity. In line with natural rhythms and cycles, each doṣa governs a time of day, of month, a season, and time of life. Knowing when each doṣa is dominant can give us insight into which qualities to be aware of and when, and how to use the qualities of a particular doṣa to our advantage. This is a helpful tool for maintaining health and balance, and for preventing dis-ease.

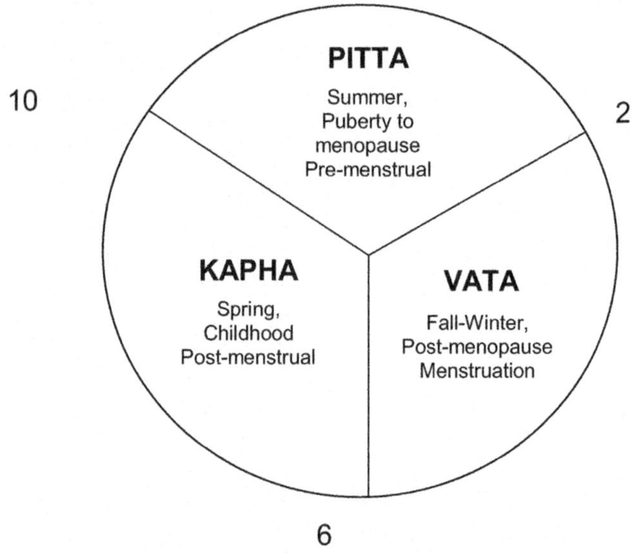

Information that I found helpful about this cycle comes from John Douillard's book *The 3-Season Diet: Eat the Way Nature Intended*.[108] I appreciate how he outlines the physiological

108 Dr. John Douillard, *The 3-Season Diet* (New York: Three Rivers Press, 2000), 155.

specifics of the cycles and how they can be most effectively used for our wellness. Under the ***physiological impact of qualities*** section, I have added in parentheses which guṇas[109] are dominant at that time of day.

Dominant Doṣa	Time[110]	Physiological Impact of Qualities
Kapha	6 a.m. - 10 a.m.	Muscles get stronger (↑ in the stable and gross guṇas)
Pitta	10 a.m. - 2 p.m.	Digestion gets stronger (↑ in hot and sharp guṇas)
Vāta	2 p.m. - 6 p.m.	Nervous system activates (↑ in the subtle guṇa)
Kapha	6 p.m. - 10 p.m.	Metabolism slows for sleep (↑ in the heavy and dull guṇas)
Pitta	10 p.m. - 2 a.m.	Liver is activated for cleansing (↑ in the sharp and clear guṇas)
Vāta	2 a.m. - 6 a.m.	Cortisol levels increase (↑ in the light and mobile guṇas)

Based on how our bodies respond to the doṣic rhythms, certain activities are better performed at different times, specifically:

1. Wake before sunrise, when the body is lightest.
2. Exercise in the morning, when the body is strongest.
3. Eat your biggest meal at lunch, when digestion is strongest.

109 If you're ever unsure, come back to the guṇas!

110 The times are approximate in the sense that there is variation based on seasons.

Do you notice how each of these Āyurvedic recommendations uses the guṇas of a doṣa to our advantage for health? We use the light guṇa of *vāta* to help us get going in the morning, the stability of *kapha* for exercise (very demanding activity!), and the sharp hot nature of *pitta* to digest better. Isn't the system brilliant? This is what it means to *align with the rhythms of nature*—we follow the flow of nature, and health follows.

CHAPTER 12

VĀTA DOṢA: AIR + ETHER

Vāta is a combination of the air and ether elements. As a result, it embodies the following guṇas[111]:

1. Dry (*rūkṣa*)
2. Light (*laghu*)
3. Cold (*śīta*)
4. Rough (*khara*)
5. Subtle (*sūkṣma*)
6. Mobile (*cala*)
7. Clear (*viśada*)

Given what we already know about the guṇas, we can understand why to balance *vāta* doṣa we want to keep the following qualities and ideas at the forefront of everything we offer:

Stable
Warm
Calm
Grounded
Soothed
Nourished
Peaceful
Slow

111 From the *Aṣṭāṅga Hṛdayam*, *Sūtrasthāna* 1.11.

Biology and Physiology Governed by *Vāta*

Vāta is considered the "King of the Doṣas" because it is "that which moves." This means that anywhere in the body-mind where there is movement—from neural impulses to muscular contractions to the ingestion of nourishment to the elimination of wastes—*vāta* is there to move it. The other two doṣas are considered lame—they do not move without *vāta's* support. This is a big job in a system that is in constant motion!

Vāta's main functions are:

- Maintains life—is the **key** for the physical body / physiology
- Catabolic (degenerative)
- Centrifugal (dispersive)
- Initiates mental activities (*manas*)
- Moderates the senses (*indriyas*)
- Organizes the tissues (*dhātu*)
- Coordinates the body
- Responsible for communication
- Root of pleasure and enthusiasm
- Stimulates digestive fire (*agni*)
- Dehydrates and dries up the doṣas
- Eliminates the excretory products (*malas*)
- Forms spaces and cavities in the body (*śārīra*)

Vāta governs the following organs and organ systems:

- **Colon**—primary site of *vāta* (its home)
- Urinary-bladder, rectum and pelvis
- Waist, thighs, and legs
- Bones—all of the skeletal tissues, the sacrum in particular
- Ears and skin
- Brain and nervous system

Seasonal Effects on *Vāta*

1. ***Accumulation:*** *Vāta* begins to accumulate in the late summer since the digestive fire is weaker and the body's water levels are low due to perspiration. The dry and light qualities of the summer are dominant in nature and food, which increase *vāta* in the body-mind. The heat of summer keeps *vāta* from being excessive.
2. ***Aggravation:*** *Vāta* aggravates in the late fall and early winter, as the cold and dry qualities become dominant.

   The early actions to reduce aggravation include:

   - Oleation (*snehana*)
   - Sweat therapy (*svedana*)
3. ***Alleviation:*** *Vāta* reduction occurs naturally in the spring as the humidity and heat increase in the environment.

Balancing *Vāta* Doṣa through Yoga

A note on trauma sensitivity: I mentioned at the beginning of the book that my student base has invited me to learn about teaching Yoga in a trauma-informed way. From an Āyurvedic perspective, when someone has trauma, the amount of *vāta* in their system goes up (the more trauma, the more *vāta*), creating an imbalance. Although it tends to be good form in Āyurvedic Yoga to pay attention to *vāta* at all times while teaching and practicing, I would say that teaching those with trauma involves working with *vāta* all the time, likely even choosing to balance *vāta* over other factors (like season, stage of life, etc.).

Āsana

Pace: *Vāta* can go all over the place, due to its mobile nature, which when excessive can become erratic. Where we can use the practice to create a stable structure, *vāta* settles. Use a consistent and steady pace during practice to create this stability. *Vāta* also tends to be hard and move fast, so where we can offer a practice that slows *vāta* down and invites softness, *vāta* finds more balance.

Regular practice: *Vāta's* erratic nature is balanced through consistency and containership, which increases the stable quality—one of the things *vāta* needs most. One of the best ways we can do this is through a regular practice, preferably daily, and at the same time each day if possible. You can use a set sequence per season so you don't have to figure out what to practice.

Use closed-chain postures: This means that both ends of the

pose are firmly grounded. Examples include tabletop-based poses like *Durga-Go* (Cat-Cow) and *Adho Mukha Śvānāsana* (Downward Facing Dog). These types of poses enable us to use the bones for support to avoid overworking the muscles. It also gives more points of contact with the earth, which increases the stable quality and a sense of grounding and support.

Emphasize a practice that promotes warming, circulation, and downward movement of energy (*apāna vāyu*): The tendency for *vāta* balancing is to get people to lie down and put blankets on them. This is opposite of its mobile quality for sure. Yet, have you ever noticed that this approach rarely works? Since the nature of *vāta* is mobility, an approach that feels more natural to a *vāta* type is to channel the movements with structure to bring in more stability. Encourage movement that is grounding and stabilizing, that warms the body (lying on the floor gets cold) and circulates the warmth to the periphery. Keywords: Slow flow. One of my favourite *vāta* flows is *Go* (Cow) into *Adho Mukha Śvānāsana* (Downward Facing Dog). Another is *Utthita Tāḍāsana* (Extended Mountain) into *Utkaṭāsana* (Chair). If you repeat these mindfully and with *Ujjāyī prāṇāyāma*, the *prāṇa* regulates beautifully and flows smoothly. Once the flow of *prāṇa* is regulated and the body warmed, then you can do some Restorative Yoga.

Focus on moving the *prāṇa* (breath) into the seat of *vāta* (the low belly and pelvis): In each posture, invite the inhalation into the bowl of the pelvis, into the legs, and into the soles of the feet. This is deeply nourishing (which *vāta* needs, given its catabolic tendencies) and very grounding. This breathing pattern also supports *apāna vāyu*, the downward and grounded movement of *prāṇa*.

Use ample standing postures, seated postures, forward folds, and hip openers: Make sure the energy flows down through the legs and to the feet; this is best accomplished using standing poses. Since *vāta* governs the bones, we want to use the bones as we practice. Seated postures bring the bowl of the pelvis into contact with the earth, which gives a sense of grounding and stability. Forward folds calm the nervous system, also governed by *vāta* doṣa. And finally, hip openers, especially ones that offer strong compression of the femur in the hip socket—think *Kapotāsana* (Pigeon)—are great to move excess *vāta* out of the pelvis, which is the home or seat of *vāta*, and where it builds up first.

Focus on longer, warmer, heavier integration (10 to 20 mins): The integration portion of the practice is useful for calming the nervous system, which is governed by *vāta*. Taking more time in integration (whether you choose *Śavāsana* or *Viparīta Karaṇī*) increases the slow and stable qualities. Making sure you are warm enough, with the use heavy blankets, increases the hot, heavy, and dense qualities.

Offer gentle and compassionate touch: *Vāta* types are responsive to touch (the sense that relates to the air element) and gentle touch is helpful to soothe fear and anxiety, which happens when *vāta* is high. Downward presses provide support, compression, and a sense of grounding. Compassionate touch increases the hot and oily qualities, balancing *vāta's* cold and dry nature.

If you are working with folks who have trauma, it is important to ask before touching. The surprise of unexpected touch can trigger someone's trauma, especially if the trauma was based in unwanted touch.

Prāṇāyāma

Focus on moving the *prāṇa* (breath) into the seat of *vāta* (the low belly and pelvis): This nourishes *apāna vāyu*, which stabilizes all the other sub-doṣas of *vāta*. It also promotes a sense of grounding and stability, useful for *vāta* types or in *vāta* seasons.

Emphasize the inhalation: The inhalation is the part of the breath that is nourishing (oxygenating) and filling. Focusing on this part of the breath promotes a sense of fullness and nourishment, which balances the empty and void qualities of the ether element. When we pause in our breath, any retention is an extension of whatever came before it. So to increase the sense of nourishment and fullness, you can add a pause after the inhalation.

Slow and even *Ujjāyī* (Victorious or Ocean Sounding Breath): This helps to warm the body, circulate the *prāṇa* and fluids, and calm the mind and emotions.

Nāḍī Śodhana (Alternate Nostril Breath): This is considered "good at all times" according to Dr. Scott Blossom. This technique calms the nervous system, stabilizes the mind, and purifies the subtle *prāṇic* channels, which are all beneficial for balancing *vāta* doṣa.

Meditation

Take 10 to 30 minutes to meditate: Meditation is beneficial for calming the nervous system, and therefore *vāta* doṣa. To balance *vāta*, the recommendation is to meditate after *āsana* practice, once the *prāṇa* has been reorganized to flow smoothly. I find it takes at least 10 minutes to settle *vāta* in order to actually get into a meditative state.

If imagery is part of your meditation practice, bring in **grounding, warming, and nurturing** imagery.

Yoga Nidrā: This is a very effective meditation technique to balance *vāta* doṣa. It uses the sense of hearing,[112] which is connected to *vāta*, to maintain the attention and focus of the practitioner. Instead of getting lost in silence, the steady and consistent guidance of the voice keeps the practice flowing and moving in the direction of integration. Yoga Nidrā can be a very restorative practice, which is useful and balancing for nervous, anxious, and overwhelmed *vāta*.

Trāṭaka (steady gazing): Steadying the focus, especially if it's on a warm flame, is very stabilizing and warming for *vāta*. Again, consistency, stability, and warmth are key to helping *vāta* find balance.

Mantra

Mantra Japa (Repetition): The *vāta* mind tends to be very active, and *mantra* repetition is the mental equivalent to "slow flow." Here we use *mantra* to guide the mind in a particular way, eventually creating stability and support through the

112 Air moving through space.

sound and effect of the *mantra*. It is useful to pacify an active mind.

Vāta needs soothing and protective *mantras*. Some examples include:

- Seed sounds of aim, hum, shreem/sham, ram, hrim[113]
- *Bīja Mantras* of "laṃ" (earth), "vaṃ" (water), and "raṃ" (fire)
- The Green *Tārā Mantra* "Om tare tutare ture so ha" is soothing, nurturing, and protective

Focus

Having a set and steady focal point is helpful in reducing the mobile quality. Using a focal point on the floor helps reduce the light quality. Keeping the same focal point for the practice supports stability (reducing mobility and erratic qualities). I also like to use the seat of *vāta* (bowl of the pelvis) as a focal point, and the bones too (*vāta* areas and tissues).

Language

Using a soft and steady tone balances the hard and erratic qualities of *vāta*.

113 Gary Gran, "Ayurveda & Mantra, Part 2," *Yoga Chicago* (website), July 13, 2018, http://yogachicago.com/2014/03/ayurveda-mantra-part-2/.

Colours

Earthy dark warm colours help balance *vāta* doṣa—black, charcoal, brown, rust, maroon, dark red, burgundy, and burnt orange.

Menstruation and Vāta

The menstrual cycle is an important aspect of a woman's health. I grew up in a culture with menses being seen as "the curse," or even more strangely "Aunt Flo." Talk about a way to disembody and disengage from this useful and powerful process.

For most women, the menstrual cycle follows a pattern of releasing tissues, toxins, and energy from the body about once every twenty-eight to forty days. This release is governed by *vāta* doṣa, specifically the aspect of *vāta* doṣa known as *apāna vāyu*. *Apāna vāyu* is the downward and outward moving flow. Not only does *apāna* govern menstruation, it also governs urination, defecation, and childbirth. An important aspect of *vāta* indeed!

Have you ever heard the caution in a yoga class about "not doing inversions during the moon cycle"? Supporting the natural direction of *apāna vāyu*'s flow is why. When *apāna* engages to move things "down and out" from the body as part of a natural biological cycle (e.g., daily bowel movements, daily urinations, monthly menstruation), we want to support this natural flow. Holding an inversion during menses, whether *Adho Mukha Śvānāsana* (Downward Facing Dog) or *Śīrṣāsana* (Headstand), creates a situation where gravity is going against the natural flow, and this is not good for our health and well-being.

There isn't always much thought given to the importance of menstruation, nor to the self-care that is useful during this time. It is a time when the body and energies are very busy and working hard—a time of shedding tissues no longer needed to make space for the possibility of new growth, a time of releasing wastes from the body to keep our channels clear and open, an opportunity to connect to the deep wisdom that resides within us if we're willing to turn inward.

From the Āyurvedic view, when the body has this much work going on, we create balance in the system by taking rest. How we approach this is unique to each woman, and it depends on her needs and her specific situation. Generally, when the flow is heaviest, Āyurveda recommends women rest and take a break from vigorous practice, including *āsana* and *prāṇāyāma*. An option that has worked well for me, as I appreciate the stability and consistency of a daily practice, is to continue my meditation practice, or to choose a supported restorative yoga pose [like *Sālamba Supta Baddha Koṇāsana* (Supported Reclined Bound Angle)] and enjoy a Yoga Nidrā. When the flow lightens, I might add a short gentle practice with gentle *prāṇāyāma*, like Diaphragmatic Breathing or *Nāḍī Śodhana*.

As mentioned above, many women struggle with their menstrual cycles. Painful menstruation is a sign of imbalance in the body-mind—it is not the normal flow of things. If you find yourself in this situation and want it to change, consider finding a health care provider to support you. In my personal experience, Āyurvedic health counsellors and naturopathic doctors are amazing in this realm—especially if they have a focus on women's health.

For those who are still resisting the possibility of honouring their menstrual cycle, this significant sign of health for a woman, I recommend two books to all my clients (and I buy the first one for any teenager in my life!):

1. *Reflections of the Moon on Water* by Xiaolan Zhao, CMD. It's a book about women's health, and it was the first book that invited me to think of my menstruation as something other than a curse. If I were the Empress of the Universe, I would gift this to everyone with a female biology.
2. *Balance your Hormones, Balance your Life* by Dr. Claudia Welch, MSOM. This is another fantastic book on women's health that includes a strong *Āyurvedic* perspective.

Āyurveda has taught me that if I pay attention to my menstrual cycle it will let me know how I'm doing. Am I managing my stress well? Am I eating well? Am I sleeping well? Are my emotions building up? Am I doing too much? For women, any disturbance in our system will make itself known, especially during the menstrual cycle. Although painful and difficult menses have been normalized (and hidden—Advil, anyone?), it does not have to be this way. This is our body telling us that something is up, and our attention is required.

Sample Class to Balance *Vāta* Doṣa

Music: something ambient with few lyrics (if any at all)

Setup:

1. 2 blocks
2. 2 tadpoles (which are like mini bolsters)
3. 2 blankets
4. 2 belly bags
5. 1 eye pillow
6. Anything else for comfort in integration

Opening/Centering		
	Sukhāsana/Vīrāsana (Simple Seat)	Grounding Intention setting
Prāṇāyāma		
	Nāḍī Śodhana (Alternate Nostril Breathing)	
***Āsana*—crouching**		****Closed chain poses**
	Table Top	"**Feel** the palms of the hands, and the shins **rooting** into the **earth.**"
	Durgā-Go Vinyāsa (Cat-Cow flow) *Bālāsana* (Child) into Big Back Bend	"Let the **steady breath** guide the **rhythmic** movement."
	Leg Stretch Alternate Arm & Leg Lift	
	Bhagerāsana Vinyāsa (Tiger flow) Lunge flow w hamstring stretch *Ardha Ustrāsana* (Half-Camel) R / L	

	***Āsana*—standing**	**Warming, grounding, stabilizing. Working the legs/pelvis—seat of *vāta***
	Adho Mukha Śvānāsana (Downward Facing Dog)	
	Uttānāsana (Standing Forward Fold)	
	Tāḍāsana (Mountain)	
	Sūrya Prāṇāyāma Vinyāsa (Packing the *Prāṇa*)	Engages *apāna vāyu*
	Daśa calana (Churnings) Ankles Neck Shoulders Wrists Thoracic twist Hips Knees Spinal Wave	Warming, lubricating, calming
	Ayetāsana (Goat)	Grounding, stabilizing, calming
	Vṛkṣāsana (Tree) Stargazer (Warrior 1 var) *Vīrabhadrāsana 1 Vinyāsa* (Warrior 1 flow) *Garuḍāsana* (Eagle) R / L	Grounding, stabilizing, warming
	Prasārita Pādottānāsana (Wide-Legged Forward Fold) Lateral flow (R & L) *Prasārita Adho Mukha Śvānāsana* (Wide-legged dog)	Grounding, stabilizing, calming
	Mālāsana (Squat)	

***Āsana*—reclined**		
	Supta Pavanmuktāsana (Reclined Knee to Chest) R & L	Working the legs/pelvis—seat of *vāta*
	Setu Bandhāsana (*bridge*)	Working the legs/pelvis—seat of *vāta*
	Windshield wipers (knees side to side w feet wide) *Supta Jaṭhara Parivṛttāsana* (Reclined Spinal Twist)	Working the legs/pelvis—seat of *vāta*
Integration		
	Śavāsana (Corpse) OR CRP (Constructive Rest Pose) OR *Viparīta Karaṇī* (Legs Up the Wall)	Longer duration Warm—blankets Heavy & grounding—Bean bags
Meditation & *Mantra*		
	Yoga Nidrā	Consistent pacing. Focus on warmth, heaviness, points of contact with the earth (grounding), smooth flow of breath, and feeling nourished by the practice.

CHAPTER 13

PITTA DOṢA: FIRE + WATER

Pitta is a combination of the fire and water elements. As a result, it embodies the following Guṇas[114]:

1. Oily (*sneha*)
2. Sharp/penetrating (*tīkṣṇa*)
3. Hot (*uṣṇa*)
4. Light (*laghu*)
5. Fleshy smelling (*visraṃ*)
6. Spreading (*sara*)
7. Liquid (*drava*)

Given what we already know about the guṇas, we can understand why to balance *pitta* doṣa we want to keep the following qualities and ideas at the forefront of everything we offer:

Cool
Non-Competitive
Soft
Balanced
Expansion for ventilation
Relaxing
Quiet
Surrender

114 From the *Aṣṭāṅga Hṛdayam, Sūtrasthāna* 1.12.

Biology and Physiology Governed by *Pitta*

Each doṣa governs a specific set of functions, and *pitta's* energy is "that which digests things"—from food to thoughts and emotions or experiences—*pitta* is the power of digestion and transformation in the body.

Pitta's main functions are:

- Good digestion
- Metabolism (transformation)
- Ability to taste your food
- Body temperature regulation
- Good vision
- Production of hunger, thirst, appetite
- Suppleness of the body
- Complexion
- Lustre of the eyes, hair, skin
- Happiness
- Intelligence and understanding
- Ambition and bravery

Pitta governs the following organs and organ systems:

- Lower part of the stomach and small intestine—primary site of *pitta* (its home)
- Liver, gallbladder, spleen, and pancreas
- Blood
- Eyes
- Gray matter of the brain
- Sweat glands and skin

Seasonal Effects on *Pitta*

1. ***Accumulation:*** *Pitta* begins to accumulate from spring to summer due to the change from cool and dry to hot and damp—*pitta* is warm and moist in nature.
2. ***Aggravation:*** As the summer becomes hotter, *pitta* will aggravate.

   The early actions to reduce aggravation include:

   - Oleation (snehana)—with a cooling oil[115]
   - Herbal steam bath (svedana)—less hot
   - Head oleation (śīrodhara) with cooling herbs

3. ***Alleviation:*** *Pitta* reduction occurs naturally in the fall as the temperatures cool down and the environment becomes drier in nature.

Balancing *Pitta* Doṣa through Yoga

Āsana

Teach a cooling, non-competitive, relaxing practice: Given that *pitta* is governed by the fire element, the hot, sharp, penetrating, and intense qualities are aplenty! We balance these through a cooling practice that is non-competitive[116] and cultivates ease to balance *pitta's* natural intensity. The heat and intensity of *pitta* puts folks with a predominance of

115 Like coconut or ghee. Āyurveda has a brilliant system of classification based on guṇas for all substances. It's very useful.

116 Dull instead of sharp.

these qualities at risk of burnout, so resting is important to keep them healthy and balanced.

Work with the eyes closed to encourage inward focus: The eyes are governed by *pitta*,[117] so closing the eyes does two things: 1) it allows this sense organ to relax and rest, and 2) it keeps *pitta* from looking around and getting intense and/or competitive.[118] Instead, the invitation is for *pitta* to look inward and see where they are at and what they need.

Practice in creative ways that encourage intuitive reflection instead of comparison or competition: *Pitta's* natural intensity leads to competition, which can lead to judgment and criticism. This is not good for *pitta* or anyone else. Instead, inviting *pitta* to take that sharp and penetrating capacity to self-reflect, their intelligence to intuit, provides the opportunity to use the gifts of *pitta* in a healthy, supportive, and inspired capacity.

Avoid creating too much heat: *Pitta's* connection to the fire element puts it at risk of overheating and the accompanying negative side effects. A cooling practice is very important for the *pitta* types, especially keeping the head and guts cool. Along this line, I'm going to mention that Hot Yoga is not great for *pitta* types,[119] especially in the *pitta* season.[120] *Pittas* do better with an outdoor practice in nature during the summertime.

117 Related to the fire element.

118 Or if you're really *pitta* dominant, both!

119 Even if people dislike me as a result.

120 hot + hot + hot = spontaneous combustion

Laughter Yoga: This type of practice challenges *pitta* in a new and creative way. It invites them to have fun, to relax, be playful, and surrender control and intellect,[121] which is balancing to their intense nature.

Practice during the cooler times of day: A lunch hour practice tends to adversely affect pitta's digestive capacity, and increases the tendency to overheat the body. Where *pitta* can practice in the morning (before the sun gets too hot) or in the evening (as the sun goes down), *pitta* will have more success cooling down and finding balance.

Incorporate Moon Salutations, twists, straight-legged poses (especially standing), and forward bends that stretch the inner and outer legs: The cooling nature of Moon Salutations is ideal for *pitta*. Also, doing something different satisfies the craving for something that engages their mind.[122] Twists help to wring the heat out of the digestive organs,[123] therefore, twisting postures are useful to balance *pitta*. Standing straight-legged poses are more cooling than bent-knee poses,[124] so choosing *Trikoṇāsana* (Triangle) over *Pārśvakoṇāsana* (Side Angle), or Five-Pointed Star over *Deviāsana* (Goddess) will keep the heat of *pitta* at bay. Forward bends are generally cooling,[125] and if done with the legs wide then the heat gets to ventilate out through the inner legs (groin area). Another area of the body that heat likes to move out from is the underarms, so using

121 The *pitta* person's armor of choice.

122 They love to learn new things!

123 Seat of *pitta* doṣa.

124 Think chair versus mountain: Which one is more heating?

125 Known to calm the nervous system.

goal post arms or keeping the arms at shoulder height allows more heat to leave the body.

Use parasympathetic-inducing poses: Calming postures, like *Sālamba Matsyāsana* (Supported Fish) and *Viparīta Karaṇī* (Legs Up the Wall), are very helpful for *pitta* doṣa. *Pittas* need to support and nurture the delicate (and often overused) tissues of the heart and brain. In Āyurveda, the heart-mind are one field of awareness, as opposed to separate organs. The heart in particular is adversely affected by heat.

Use medium-length cooling integration (7 to 12 mins): *Pittas* need a cooler integration. If using *Śavāsana*, have them spread out more so the heat can leave the body through the groin and armpits. This is why *Sālamba Supta Baddha Koṇāsana* (Supported Reclined Bound Angle) also works well for *pitta*—the places that need space to air out can in this pose, yet they are still fully supported and able to rest. With *pitta* types, you won't need heavy blankets. Don't worry about them getting cold—they would love it if that happened.

Prāṇāyāma

Emphasize relaxing during exhalation: The exhalation is the surrendering part of the breath, and surrendering is important for balancing the intensity of *pitta*.

Focus on rooting the breath at the navel, which is the seat of *pitta*: Use the breath to air out the hot digestive organs. Abdominal breathing provides this opportunity. Not airing out the heat causes a buildup, and this increases *pitta* imbalance.

Focus on smooth, slow, rhythmic breath: Even out the inhalations and exhalations—balance is key to *pitta*. *Pitta* tends to be extreme, going to one end of the continuum or the other. *Pitta* also tends toward intensity (hot, sharp, penetrating). Smooth, slow, rhythmic breaths are *pitta*-balancing for two reasons: 1) better aeration (move excess heat out) and 2) to stabilize *agni* (the digestive potential). *Pitta* and *agni* have a powerful relationship: as *pitta* increases, *agni* decreases. This is not a good thing because *agni* is the positive and health-promoting manifestation of the fire element, whereas *pitta* (being a doṣa) is the disease-provoking manifestation of the fire element, especially if it is out of balance.

Use cooling breaths: Cooling breaths release heat from the body, skin, emotions, and mind. Examples of cooling breaths include *Śītalī*, *Śītakarī*, and sighing.

Meditation

Focus on cooling, watery, moonlight, and relaxing imagery: Use these images if visualization is part of your concentration practice.

Use *Metta* Meditation (loving kindness): This is a wonderful meditation to transform anger, resentment, and/or hatred. *Pitta* tends to lean on the mind, and so a meditation that moves energy through the heart is very balancing and offers *pitta* a different kind of challenge. Focus is not a problem for *pitta* types, staying cool and calm is the challenge.

Explore Open Palm Meditation: This is a practice of being in your body and surrendering wilfulness—exactly what *pitta* must master to stay healthy, balanced, and strong.

Mantra

Pitta needs cooling and calming *mantras*. Some examples include:

- Seed sounds of hrim, ah, som, sham/shreem, shum, aim[126]
- *Bīja Mantras* of "laṃ" (earth), "yaṃ" (air), and "haṃ" (ether)
- *Soma Mantras* like "Om Som Somaya Namaha" and "Om Eem Shreem Somaya Namaha" are cooling and lunar
- *Guru Mantra* encouraging surrender to the teacher
- "*So Haṃ*" calms the breath and mind

Focus

Inward focus is mentioned above.

Language

Precision, clarity, and expertise are very important to *pitta* types. They will not relax[127] in a class if they do not feel the teacher is up to the task. Instead they will think they should be teaching the class and will try to figure out the best way to take over.

Colours

Cool calming colours: white, blue, green, and pastels.

---

126 Gary Gran, "Ayurveda & Mantra, Part 2."

127 I.e., surrender.

Sample Class to Balance *Pitta* Doṣa

Music: ambient with NO lyrics

Setup:

1. 2 blocks
2. 1 strap
3. 1 tadpole
4. 1 eye bag
5. Anything else for comfort in integration

Opening/Centering		
	Sukhāsana/Vīrāsana (Simple Seat)	Set intention
Prāṇāyāma		
	Dirgha Prāṇāyāma (2/3-Part Breath) Balancing inhalations w exhalations Focus on soft and easeful	Aerating Breath (venting)
***Āsana*—crouching**		
	Table Top	"**Focus** on the **sensation** of length through the spine as you inhale, and **strength** through the waistline on exhalations." Precision, inward focus
	Durgā-Go Vinyāsa (Cat-Cow flow) Cow into *Adho Mukha Śvānāsana* (Downward Facing Dog) *Adho Mukha Śvānāsana* into Big Back Bend	

	Adho Mukha Śvānāsana (Downward Facing Dog) to Core Plank *Vinyāsa* Center (knee to chest) Outer (knee to armpit) Inner (knee to opposite arm) *Kapotāsana* (Pigeon) Sunbird *Bālāsana* (Child) R & L	Working the abdomen in various ways (seat of *pitta*) Venting of armpits and legs Embedding resting poses **Pitta* will not be "satisfied" if they don't feel like they've "worked" ☺
***Āsana*—standing**		
	Uttānāsana (Standing Forward Fold)	
	Tāḍāsana (Mountain)	
	Candra Namaskar variation (Moon Salutations): *Candrāsana Vinyāsa* (Half Moon flow R & L) *Anjayenāsana* (Lunge) into flow w *Pārśvottānāsana* (Pyramid Leg Stretch) *Trikoṇāsana* (Triangle) *Ardha Candrāsana* (Half Moon Balance) Five-Pointed Star *Deviāsana* (Goddess) + twist *Tāḍāsana* (Mountain) R & L	Expansive, aerating, precise Many straight-legged standing poses Working the abdominals (*agni* stoking) Balancing poses and complex transitions to offer challenge
	Prasārita Pādottānāsana (Wide-Legged Forward Fold) *Prasārita Adho Mukha Śvānāsana* (Wide-Legged Dog) Runners Stretch (side to side)	Aerating, wide straight legs
	Baddha Koṇāsana balance (Bound Angle Toe Squat)	

***Āsana*—seated**		
	Vakrāsana (Seated Spinal Twist) *Jānu Śīrṣāsana* (Head to Knee)	Twisting to wring out excess *pitta* *Jānu* vents through the groin
Prāṇāyāma		
	Śītalī OR *Śītakarī Prāṇāyāma* (Cooling Breath)	Cooling
***Āsana*—reclined**		
	Supta Pavanmuktāsana (Reclined Knee to Chest) Hamstring stretch *Jaṭhara Parivrittāsana* with Straight-Legs R & L	
	Salamba Sarvāṅgāsana (Supported Shoulderstand)	Relaxing, easeful, cooling, not competitive, and rejuvenative
	Windshield Wipers (knees side to side w feet wide) *Supta Jaṭhara Parivṛttāsana* (Reclined Spinal Twist)	
	Śavāsana (Corpse)	Medium length Cooling—lighter or no blankets Eye bag to soothe the eyes Spread the legs and arms
Meditation & *Mantra*		
	Metta Meditation (loving kindness)	

CHAPTER 14

KAPHA DOṢA: WATER + EARTH

Kapha is a combination of the water and earth elements. Since these are the most substantial of the elements, you might notice that *kapha* has more guṇas than the other doṣas. It embodies the following guṇas[128]:

1. Oily (*snigdha*)
2. Cool (*śīta*)
3. Heavy (*guru*)
4. Slow (*manda*)
5. Smooth (*ślakṣṇa*)
6. Soft (*mṛdu*)
7. Stable (*sthira*)
8. Dense (*sāndra*)
9. Cloudy (*piccila*)
10. Gross/Big/Obvious (*sthūla*)

Given what we already know about the guṇas, we can understand why to balance *kapha* doṣa, we want to keep the following qualities and ideas at the forefront of everything we offer:

---

128 From the *Aṣṭāṅga Hṛdayam, Sūtrasthāna* 1.12.

Stimulate

Warm

Uplift

Happy

Energize

Moving

Activate

Biology and Physiology Governed by *Kapha*

Kapha is the energy of nourishment and cohesion. It is responsible for the entire structure of our biology and its ability to use nourishment to sustain itself.

Kapha's main functions are:

- Cohesion (things coming together)
- Anabolic (growth promoting)
- Stability (commitment)
- Heaviness
- Unctuousness
- Immunity—white blood cells and lymph
- Fertility / Reproduction (virility)—semen is a *kapha* tissue
- Strength, patience and forbearance—can handle things
- Fortitude (inner strength—mental and emotional)
- Benevolence (goodwill)
- Loving

Kapha governs the following organs and organ systems:

- Chest—the primary site of *kapha* doṣa is the *hṛdaya* (lungs and heart)
- Upper stomach
- Tongue and mouth
- Head and brain
- Joints
- Adipose tissue

Seasonal Effects on *Kapha*

1. ***Accumulation:*** *Kapha* begins to accumulate with the onset of winter and its cool qualities. Heavier foods are eaten in the winter, which can also accumulate *kapha*.
2. ***Aggravation:*** *Kapha* aggravates in the spring, as the heat liquefies accumulated *kapha* (mucous).

   Early actions to reduce aggravation include:

   - Oleation (*snehana*)—internal and external
   - Herbal steam bath (*svedana*)
   - Herbal paste and oil application (*udvartana*)
3. ***Alleviation:*** *Kapha* reduction occurs naturally in the summer with its light, dry, and hot qualities.

Balancing *Kapha* Doṣa through Yoga

Āsana

Use a gradual and step-by-step manner: *Kapha* must be moved into a more vigorous practice in a gradual and step-by-step manner, not just told to move more. The heaviness of *kapha* must be coaxed into movement. The tendency is to want to move them "fast and hard," like an aerobics class; however, *kapha* can be stubborn, and that doesn't always work. Once that *kapha* ball gets rolling, *kapha* will happily keep on moving. *Kapha* types have the best endurance of all the doṣas.

Kapha requires awakening on all levels: This means a practice that is more than physical. Create a practice that includes the senses, breath, imagination, emotions, and spiritual realms. The more aspects you can bring into the practice, the more interested *kapha* will be, and the more participation you will see.

Practice in the morning: Since the morning is governed by *kapha*,[129] it is important that *kapha* moves in the morning to keep things from stagnating[130] in the body-mind.

Emphasize a practice that is active and warming: Include *Sūrya Namaskār* (Sun Salutations), fluid *Vinyāsas*, squats, standing forward and backbends, and warming inversions.[131]

---

129 From 6 a.m. to 10 a.m.: the heavy, stable, and thick qualities increase.

130 Think coagulation.

131 Like Headstand and Forearm Balance.

Mindful *Vinyāsa* is ideal for cool *kapha* doṣa—flow, movement, warmth, and circulation. *Kapha* is known for its endurance and it benefits from movement to cultivate a sense of lightness, warmth, and expansiveness.

Remember that effort does not equal *kapha* reduction: To reduce *kapha*, it is necessary to protect the balance of *vāta* while practicing. Excessive muscular effort obstructs the proper flow of *vāta* through the channels and disrupts the nervous system. The body will try to stabilize the disruption and instability by creating more *kapha*.

Prāṇāyāma

Focus on moving the *prāṇa* (breath) into the seat of *kapha* (the chest and ribs): Emphasize thoracic breathing. Bring more air element into the seat of *kapha* (chest) as a way to balance the system overall. The light dryness of the air in the lungs is helpful to balance the heavy stickiness of *kapha*. That said, let's not forget to keep *vāta* pacified by taking some breaths into the lower belly and pelvis as needed.

Emphasize deep, full breaths: To keep fluid from building up in the lungs,[132] I invite my students to inhale and fill the whole torso like a balloon then to exhale and squeeze all the air out. The exhalation is the *kapha*-balancing part of the breath because it is "empty" and hollow—the opposite of *kapha's* fullness. Adding a slight pause after the exhalation promotes more of the space element, which balances *kapha's* earth element qualities.

---

132 The seat of *kapha*, which means the place it likes to build up or accumulate.

Smooth and rhythmic *Ujjāyī* (Victorious): This helps to warm the body and circulate the *prāṇa* and fluids.

Try *Kapālabhāti* and *Bhastrikā*: These are excellent for melting excess *kapha* in the chest and head, provided it does not disturb *pitta* or *vāta*. These breaths are lightening (reducing) and invigorating, which is a great balance to *kapha's* heavy, dense, thick, stickiness.

Meditation

Explore open-eyed, standing, or walking meditations: Walking meditations keep things circulating and reduce stagnation. A great pose for standing meditation is *Ayetāsana* (Goat). Open-eyed meditation reduces the likelihood of getting sleepy (dull, thick, heavy, cloudy). Many traditions use a soft gaze instead of closed eyes for this.

If imagery is part of your meditation practice, bring in *spacious and warming* imagery.

Mantra

Kīrtan: *Kīrtan* is excellent for clearing emotional heaviness from the heart and to strengthen the lungs. It is also done in community, and that connection to others is very important to *kapha*—they love others. Being in community is stimulating, which is healthy for *kapha*.

Kapha needs stimulating and clearing *mantras*. Some examples include:

- Seed sounds of "klim," "om," "aim," "hum," "hrim"[133]

133 Gary Gran, "Ayurveda & Mantra, Part 2."

- *Bīja Mantras* of "raṃ" (fire), "yaṃ" (air), and "haṃ" (ether)
- *Gāyatrī*, "Om" and "Om Gum Ganapatayei Namaha" are powerfully clearing

Focus

Using focal points that are off the ground (think upward gaze, where the ceiling meets the wall), precise, and heart centered (image on the wall) are ideal.

Language

Light, uplifting, motivational, inspirational, and enthusiastic—all important to lift the heaviness of *kapha*.

Colours

Bright, neon, fluorescent, colourful: yellow, pink, teal, lime, fire-engine red, bright orange, neon blue.

Sample Class to Balance *Kapha* Doṣa

Music: anything uplifting, fun, motivating (lyrics!)

Setup:

1. 2 blocks
2. 1 tadpole
3. 1 eye bag
4. Anything else for comfort in integration

Centering		
	Tāḍāsana (Mountain)	Body scan Set intention
Prāṇāyāma		
	Sūrya Prāṇāyāma (Sun Breaths) w *Ujjāyī* (Victorious breath)	Fluid, warming Emphasize opening the side chest/lungs
	Dirgha Prāṇāyāma (2/3-Part Breath*)*	Emphasize opening the front chest
***Āsana*—standing**		
	Vyana Vāyu Vinyāsa Inhale into *Utthita Tāḍāsana* (Palm Tree) Exhale into *Utkaṭāsana* (Chair)	Engaging the circulating *prāṇa vāyu* (important for *kapha* doṣa)
	Ardha Candrāsana Vinyāsa (Half Moon flow)	Open the side body, including the chest
	Chest Expander *Vinyāsa* Exhale into *Utkaṭāsana* with fingers to shoulders and elbows to knees Inhale into *Tāḍāsana* w chest lifted and elbows open and wide	Opens the chest (seat of *kapha* doṣa)

	Uttānāsana (Standing Forward Fold) *Ardha Uttānāsana Vinyāsa* (Halfway Lift flow)	Inversions & flow—heat to balance, and inversion to release accumulation of *kapha*
	Anjayenāsana (Lunge) R *Vinyāsa* to *Purvottanāsana* (Pyramid to Lunge flow)	Heating as we work the legs and big muscle groups
	Vīrabhadrāsana 2 (Warrior 2) R *Pārśvakoṇāsana* to Exalted *Vira Vinyāsa* (Side Angle to Exalted Warrior flow)	Lateral bends to open the chest and strengthen the core
	Caturaṅga Daṇḍāsana (Plank) into prone (belly down)	Strengthening transition
	Uddiyanāsana (Flying Bird)	Backbends are great to move energy upward and open the chest
	Adho Mukha Śvānāsana (Downward Facing Dog)	Inversion to move release accumulation of *kapha*
	Anjayenāsana (Lunge) L *Vinyāsa* to *Purvottanāsana* (Pyramid to Lunge flow)	Heating as we work the legs and big muscle groups
	Vīrabhadrāsana 2 (Warrior 2) L *Pārśvakoṇāsana* to Exalted *Vira Vinyāsa* (Side Angle to Exalted Warrior flow)	Lateral bends to open the chest and strengthen the core
	Caturaṅga Daṇḍāsana (Plank) into prone (belly down)	Strengthening transition
	Dhanurāsana (bow)	Backbends are great to move energy upward and open the chest
	Adho Mukha Śvānāsana (Downward Facing Dog)	Inversion to move release accumulation of *kapha*

	Uttānāsana (Standing Forward Fold) *Ardha Uttānāsana Vinyāsa* (Halfway Lift flow)	Inversions & flow—heat to balance, and inversion to release accumulation of *kapha*
	Chest Expander Vinyāsa Exhale into *Utkaṭāsana* with fingers to shoulders and elbows to knees Inhale into *Tāḍāsana* w chest lifted and elbows open and wide	Opens the chest (seat of *kapha* doṣa)
	Tāḍāsana (Mountain)	
	Naṭarājāsana R & L (King Dancer)	Standing backbend to open lungs in a different way + stimulating
	Mālāsana (Squat)	Thighs parallel to keep the heat in
***Āsana*—crouching**		****Inversion series—allows for the elimination of excess *kapha***
	Forearm plank to Dolphin *Vinyāsa* Single leg lifts from Dolphin Sun Bird from Dolphin	Warming, circulating, inverting
	Anahatāsana (Melting Heart)	Inversion, chest opener
	Thread the Needle R&L	Inverted twist (wrings out the excess *kapha* and eliminates it)
	Bālāsana (Child)	Rest, mild inversion
Prāṇāyāma		
	Kapālabhāti (Shining Skull Breath)	

Āsana—reclined		
	Windshield Wipers (knees side to side w feet wide) OR *Supta Jaṭhara Parivṛttāsana* (Reclined Spinal Twist)	Unwind, release, settle
	Śavāsana (Corpse) OR *Supta Matsyāsana* (Supported Fish)	Shorter timing Warm and light Supported Fish opens the chest (seat)
Meditation & _Mantra_		
	Kīrtan (chanting)	

CHAPTER 15
CONCLUSION TO DOṢA YOGA

Contemplations for the Teacher

An important concept in the teaching of Āyurvedic Yoga is that **every doṣa can practice every pose**—how they practice the pose will determine the effect (balancing or deranging for a particular doṣa).

For the following postures, consider how you would teach them to pacify each *vāta*, *pitta*, and *kapha*:

1. *Bakāsana* (Crow)
2. *Sūrya Namaskār* (Sun Salutations)
3. *Adho Mukha Śvānāsana* (Downward Facing Dog)
4. *Tāḍāsana* (Mountain)

If you're not sure where to begin with this exercise, here are some hints:

1. Will you emphasize a different aspect of the body or posture for each of the doṣas?
2. Is it a different variation on the pose?
3. What cues make the most sense for each doṣa, given the guṇas of each doṣa?

Think about which guṇas you are going to balance for a doṣa, what are the main ideas or themes to keep in mind to balance a doṣa, and how do all those pieces fit together?

One of the Āyurvedic Yoga projects I really enjoyed was taking one class structure and modifying it to balance each of the doṣas. Here's the link to download the classes if you are interested in exploring this further: https://janatiyoga.com/?download=ayurvedic-video-lesson-bundle.

Spoiler alert: there's a code at the end of the book for a discount on the classes.

The structure of each class follows this format:

1. Centering
2. *Prāṇāyāma*
3. *Daśa Calana* (Churnings)
4. *Sūrya Namaskār* (Sun Salutations)
5. *Mālāsana* (Squat)
6. *Vakrāsana* (Seated Spinal Twist)
7. Integration in *Śavāsana* (Corpse)

As you do each practice, notice the shifts for each doṣa. Also notice if these modifications work to balance that doṣa for you.

This gives you an idea of how to use one class structure and modify it for each of the doṣas. Again, because we're focusing on the approach of teaching, it's not about picking a specific pose for a doṣa (although sometimes that makes sense too), it's really about tailoring the approach to the guṇas you want to balance, bringing us full circle to the section on Guṇa Yoga.

SECTION 3

SPECIAL TOPICS IN ĀYURVEDA

INTRODUCTION TO SPECIAL TOPICS

To me, special topics are key concepts in Āyurveda that apply to everyone regardless of doṣic or guṇa predominance. The ones I am very passionate about and want to share with you are:

1. *agni*—the digestive potential
2. *sattva*, *rajas*, and *tamas*—the doṣas of the mind
3. *ojas*—the vital protective essence

I want to be clear that this section is not going to teach you about these topics—that's what Āyurveda School[134] is for. However, for those of you who have this knowledge already, this is another way you can integrate Āyurveda into classes and/or workshops. These topics make great workshops. I've used most of them as themes for my annual Āyurvedic Yoga retreat weekend. People really enjoy diving deeper into how they can use something they enjoy (Yoga) to support themselves and find greater health (Āyurveda).

My approach is to incorporate the concepts as themes within the existing style of class I teach. Therefore, students are doing the practice while I'm teaching them in and out of poses and explaining the connection to the theme/concept as I go. That said, if I were to run a workshop on *agni*, there would be sitting/note-taking period to cover theory, then a practice component for us to experience and feel how the practice relates to the teaching.

134 And my upcoming book on Āyurveda's Three Pillars of Health being released in 2019.

Another note on *Āyurvedic* Yoga with a Trauma-Informed lens: The reason I explored these three topics in more details for classes is that, in my understanding, each of these topics relates to trauma.

- Where something really weird and/or really hard happens (trauma), our *agni* might not be able to digest the experience, leaving us with *āma* (undigested experience / trauma) in our channels—clogs in our pipes.
- When trauma causes stress to our body-mind, our *ojas* gets used up as it tries to buffer us from that stress. When this happens, we can become depleted and depressed, which makes it even more challenging to find the stability needed for healing.
- Trauma tends to move the balance of the mind into either *rajas* (agitation and fear) or *tamas* (inertia, stuckness, or depression), and creates a context where it is a challenge to find *sattva* (balance and stability). This can lead to more stress and more clogs … which potentially sets up a cycle of re-traumatization.

Working to strengthen, balance, and bring these ideas into awareness increases the likelihood that those suffering from trauma will reduce that suffering through digestion and building resilience. They will find a new equilibrium and clarity, and reconnect with their innate joy.

CHAPTER 16

AGNI: THE DIGESTIVE POTENTIAL

Agni, or inner fire, is a key concept in the Āyurvedic teachings. *Agni* is a representation of the fire element in the body-mind. It describes the biological fire, or heat energy that governs metabolism. Often, it is referred to as the *digestive fire*. Our *agni* digests our food, sensory impressions, emotions, thoughts, ideas, and experiences. Without *agni*, we are unable to use what we take into our body-minds, and whatever we cannot digest builds up as residue, known as *āma*, in our body-mind. This is why a strong *agni* is considered paramount to maintaining health. Without a strong *agni*, we end up with clogs in our pipes.

Fun fact: The first words in the Vedas around the Āyurvedic teachings are "Om Agni." This concept is so important in the Āyurvedic teachings that the teachings begin with these words! For those of you who are wondering the same thing about Yoga, the first word of Patañjali's Yoga Sūtras is "Atha," which translates to "Now" (present moment). Guess what Yoga's all about?

Back to *agni*. Caraka describes *agni* in the following ways throughout the *Caraka Saṃhitā*:[135]

> The span of life, health, immunity, energy, metabolism, complexion, strength, enthusiasm, luster, and the vital breath (prana) are all dependent on agni …

135 One of the authoritative texts on Āyurveda.

> One lives a long healthy life if it is functioning properly, becomes sick if it is deranged, or dies if this fire is extinguished . . .
>
> Proper nourishment of the body, tissues, ojas, etc., depend upon the proper functioning of agni in digestion.[136]

With this concept being so important in Āyurveda, I thought it would be both interesting and useful to design Yoga classes around *agni*. **How do we use Yoga techniques to boost and support our *agni*?**

We hear about the benefits of Yoga *āsana*, *prāṇāyāma*, *dhyāna*, and *mantra* all the time in Yoga classes, so I took all the things I knew about Yoga that were "good for digestion" and put them together in a class. Then I layered what I know about *agni* on top of that (which refined it) and created a series of *agni*-boosting classes.

These were a lot of fun. I started working on them after Thanksgiving weekend when I realized how hard the Canadian approach to Thanksgiving is on our *agni*. My students had a blast because they too were feeling the ill effects of *agni*-smothering overconsumption.

In the *agni*-boosting class explorations, I included elements like:

- ***Theory:*** What is *agni*? Why is it important? How we can use Yoga to support a strong digestive fire.

---

136 Dr. Ram Karan Sharma and Vaidya Bhagwan Dash (translations & commentaries by), *Caraka Saṃhitā* (Varanasi India: Chowkhamba Press, 2014).

- ***Guṇas:*** What are the qualities of *agni*? It is light, sharp, dry. Do we need to work on any of these qualities in particular given the season?
- ***Āsana that focuses on agni building:*** *Ayetāsana* (Goat), *Sūrya Namaskār* (Sun Salutations—the sun is *agni*!), torso rolls that focus on the abdomen, belly-down backbends, and abdominal work.[137]
- ***Āsana that focuses on apāna vāyu:*** if the inner winds are disorganized, our *agni* destabilizes. Practice poses like *Ayetāsana* (Goat), *Setu Bandhāsana* (Bridge), *Vṛkṣāsana* (Tree), *Apānāsana* (Knee to Chest), and *Prasārita Pādottānāsana* or *Uttānāsana* (Standing Forward Folds).
- ***Prāṇāyāma that focuses on agni building:*** *Kapālabhāti* (Shining Skull Breath) and *Bhastrikā* (Bellows).
- ***Prāṇāyāma that focuses on apāna vāyu:*** Diaphragmatic and *Dirgha* (2/3-Part Breath).
- ***Prāṇāyāma that focuses on samāna vāyu:*** The entire torso needs good airflow; without it, the fire cannot burn bright and strong. For this I use *Dirgha Prāṇāyāma* (2/3-Part Breath).
- ***Kriyā:*** *Uḍḍīyāna bandha kriyā*, *agni sara*, *nauli*, *akunchana prasarana* → all the gut-churning cleansing techniques are fabulous to support *agni* and *apāna vāyu*.
- ***Dhyāna:*** I believe that meditation supports the mental-emotional *agni*. I have tried a few different

137 Which might be belly-down backbends like *Bhujaṅgāsana* (Cobra/Sphinx) or core-strengthening poses like *Nāvāsana* (Boat).

techniques and continue to explore this. My favourite so far is Yoga Nidrā.

- ***Mudrā:*** agni (fire) mudrā, vāyu (air) mudrā.

When we look at it this way, we can see that there are a lot of options and the potential for many *agni*-boosting classes.

The deeper our understanding of *agni*, and how to support and stabilize *agni*, the more nuanced we can get with how we use Yoga to do this. This is one of the things I appreciate so much about Yoga and Āyurveda—the depth is unlimited and the layers of subtlety brilliant and captivating.

CHAPTER 17

SATTVA, *RAJAS*, AND *TAMAS*: THE DOṢAS OF THE MIND

Both Yoga and Āyurveda share perspective and language around working with the mind. In both sciences, the language of the mind is very specific. The language used is that of the **Mahā Guṇas**. These refer to the three "great qualities" of nature that are responsible for the creation of all substances in the world of form,[138] known as *sattva*, *rajas*, and *tamas*.

Here is a beautiful description from Patañjali's Yoga Sūtras:

> YS II.18: The object of experience is composed of the three gunas—the principles of illumination (sattva), activity (rajas), and inertia (tamas). From these, the whole universe has evolved, together with the instruments of knowledge—such as the mind, senses, etc.—and the objects perceived—such as the physical elements. The universe exists in order that the experiencer may experience it, and thus become liberated.[139]

When the mahā guṇas are in balance, we experience *sattva*—the quality of balance, calm, peace, and harmony. My meditation teacher Larry referred to this state as "relaxed alertness," the balance point between agitation and dullness.

---

138 *Prakṛti*.

139 Swami Prabhavananda and Christopher Isherwood, *How to Know God: The Yoga Aphorisms of Patanjali* (Hollywood: Vedanta Society, 1981), 130.

I think of it as awareness, the place between running away (action, agitation) and tuning out (resistance, dullness). It has an *inward and upward* movement and is the principle of *intelligence*. Many Yogis aspire to become *sattvic*, and according to the Āyurvedic teachings, we already are—we are born with a balanced, clear, and harmonious mind. What happens is that the channels of the mind get boggy, and this creates imbalance. When this happens, we experience either:

1. ***Rajas*:** Movement, enthusiasm, desire, agitation, restlessness, and false perception. *Rajas* has an outward motion and is the principle of energy.[140] It isn't *sattva* and yet it is still necessary because it is the energy needed for change and transformation.[141]
2. ***Tamas*:** Density, heaviness, darkness, dullness, ignorance, stagnation, resistance, inertia, obstruction, and lethargy. It has a downward movement and is the principle of materiality. It is most familiar in times of illness,[142] yet is needed to promote grounding, rest, and sleep.

Sattva is a positive balance between *rajas* and *tamas*. Deviation from this balance, the imbalances of *rajas* and *tamas*, are described in Āyurveda as the "doṣas of the mind."

These three qualities are in a constant ever-changing interplay, flowing from one to the next, moment to moment. The

140 All movement is *rajasic*.

141 E.g., to get from a *tamasic* state to a *sattvic* one, the energy and movement of *rajas* is necessary.

142 Lack of energy and motivation, yet not balanced and harmonious either.

practice that goes with this theory is meditation—cultivating a state of presence that allows you to recognize which mahā guṇa is active. This recognition is increasing our awareness, or boosting our *sattva*. Over time we see that each of these mahā guṇas, just like all the other guṇas, comes into being, exists, and dissolves into something else. This awareness helps us to disentangle ourselves from attachment to these guṇas, to simply experience what is flowing through our field of awareness, and let it flow.

So how do I bring this into a Yoga class? The way I've explored it so far is to explain the idea then teach the practice:

- In each technique, I have students check in with themselves—are they balanced, feeling agitated, or tuning out?
- We'll hold a posture for longer than usual—check in.
- We do a posture more quickly than usual—check in.
- While we're breathing—check in.
- While we're chanting—check in.
- Before integration—check in.
- After integration—check in.
- How do you feel about checking in?—check in.

It's been very interesting to get feedback from my students about this. Many of them come back the next week to report on what they've noticed in their own life patterns—whether they get agitated or tune out. I remind them often that noticing where they are at is cultivating balance—you can't take steps to get into balance if you don't even know you've lost your balance! Then we talk about noticing which Yoga techniques help bring in more balance, which ones agitate, when do we tune out, etc. If you're agitated or tuned out, can you use one of the balancing tools to come back to yourself in the present moment?

I've also explored *sattva, rajas* and *tamas* in a few other ways:

- If I notice that a group is more *tamasic* or dull, then we'll use a movement based practice, like *Vinyāsa* or *Dirgha Prāṇāyāma*, to stir up the inertia. David Frawley explains that we can't go from *tamas* to *sattva*—we need to use *rajas* (energy and movement) to shift the inertia.
- If what I see in a group is *rajas* or agitation, then I'll begin with gentle flows and eventually slow down to either a yin or restorative style, to bring them into conscious stillness, relaxed alertness or *sattva*. The key is to cultivate *sattva* instead of sinking them into *tamas*.
- If the group begins in a *sattvic* state, then how do we practice so that it does not create agitation, nor dullness, and instead maintains their conscious calm. Back to Goldilocks! I believe this is another meeting of the science and art of teaching—working with the energies of the mind through the body and breath practices. Working with *sattva*, *rajas*, and *tamas* can be easily connected to any of the eight limbs. There are so many great ways of exploring this concept through Yoga practice.
- We can also get technique specific, recognizing that *mantra* and *dhyāna* are designed to work with the energies of the mind. Incorporating meditation and

mantra into your classes will change whether a student lands in their *sattva*, *rajas*, or *tamas*. How we practice these techniques also matters. An example being that chanting a *mantra* loudly and quickly might agitate more than calm the mind.

There are many ways to explore Yoga tools and techniques to influence the Doṣas of the Mind. Recognizing this creates a huge potential for the use of Yoga to find more mental balance through a physical practice.

CHAPTER 18

OJAS: THE VITAL PROTECTIVE ESSENCE

Ojas is the vital protective essence and is related to vitality and immunity. It's the glue that cements the elements together to create a stable body and mind. It circulates via the heart and throughout the body to maintain the natural resistance of bodily tissues.

Ojas is a super-fine biological substance, the refined essence of all the tissues, known as *bala* (strength). *Ojas* production and maintenance is related to the proper functioning of the endocrine, nervous, skeletal, muscular, hematopoietic, and digestive systems. When all these systems perform their functions optimally, *ojas* is maintained. When a system's function goes offline,[143] our body uses *ojas* to buffer against the effects of this and any other stress.

Ojas is the container for *prāṇa*. Without *ojas*, the *prāṇa* cannot and does not stabilize.

According to Dr. David Frawley:

> [Of the three vital essences,] **the most important is Ojas**. Ojas not only gives a strong reserve of vital energy, it also provides strength and maturity of character and emotional stability. Ojas creates the vessel necessary to hold prana and tejas, which would otherwise disperse.

---

143 Becomes deranged.

> Without ojas, exercises in meditation and yoga lack the proper foundation.[144]

I have a deep resonance with this particular concept and am constantly looking for ways to build more *ojas* in my life and in my practices. I realized a few years ago that many people practice Yoga in way that depletes their *ojas*, which is why they cannot contain and stabilize their *prāṇa*. This realization reinforced my belief that these sciences are meant to be taught together; the wisdom of one deepens the wisdom of the other.

Given my obsession with *ojas*-building, this is a topic I explore often in my classes. The explorations have had many flavours and included the following:

- **Theory:** I share with the group what *ojas* is and why it's important. I tell them that *ojas* is our buffer to stress, and I invite participants to consider and notice if they are using their practice to build *ojas* or if their practice is using up their *ojas*. It is a fine line sometimes. Let's use our *sattva* to figure out where that line is so we can practice in a way that supports *ojas*.
- **Guṇas:** *Ojas* is soft, smooth, fluid/liquid, cool, and stable. I cultivate all these guṇas in an *ojas*-building class.
- ***Āsana:*** Typically, classes that are less stressful and use less energy/resources support the building of *ojas*. This includes, and yet is not limited to, styles like Restorative,

144 Dr. David Frawley, *Yoga & Ayurveda* (Twin Lakes: Lotus Press, 1999), 100.

Gentle, and Yin Yoga, and Yoga Therapy. Anything too vigorous or warming uses *ojas* instead of building it. *Ojas* is deeply connected to *brahmacharya*.[145].

- ***Prāṇāyāma:*** The ones I have worked with to build *ojas* include *Nāḍī Śodhana* (Alternate Nostril Breathing), *Brahmari* (Bumble Bee), and Mindful Breathing or Breath Awareness.
- ***Dhyāna*:** I believe that most meditation techniques are *ojas*-building. The ones I find most effective are Yoga Nidrā, *Metta* (Loving Kindness), and *Mantra Japa* (Mantra Repetition).
- ***Mantra:*** In particular *OM*, "*So Haṃ*," "*Yaṃ*," "*Om Mani Padme Hum*," and "*Asato Mā Sad Gamaya*" are considered very *ojas*-building. Because *ojas* is seated in and connected to the heart, anything done with love is *ojas*-building.
- ***Kīrtan:*** good spiritual company is *ojas*-building.
- **Intention-Setting:** My understanding of intention-setting is that we ask the wisdom embedded in our hearts[146] to share with us what it wants for us. This whisper, this heartfelt desire, is our intention. If it comes from the heart, there is a connection to *ojas*, and so setting intention from this heartfelt place is *ojas*-building too.
- **Loving Touch:** As a teacher, if you are able to connect with each student and offer loving touch or even honest and sincere praise, this also helps build their *ojas*.

---

145 The appropriate use of our vital essences of *prāṇa*, *tejas*, and *ojas*.

146 Connecting to *puruṣa* (soul).

You are probably aware that there are many ways to build *ojas* using the Yoga tools. How you want to put all these possibilities together is yours to explore.

EPILOGUE

We can use our practice to fuel one of two fires: the fire of ego or the fire of spirit.

Āyurvedic Yoga is an environmental practice—practicing based on what we see and experience in the environment. Using this method, we are not practicing based on likes and dislikes, which fuels the fire of ego, but practicing what is needed to balance our system because we recognize that we ARE nature. This clears the channels of our body-heart-mind from debris, which allows the voice of spirit to be heard. When we are connected to our spirit, we recognize not only our purpose and how to contribute to the world; we also hear the spirit of the world and how we are connected to all things. When this happens, Āyurveda becomes a practice of Spiritual Environmentalism, where we recognize that we are one with the planet, and honouring the planet is how we care for ourselves and each other. It is all one practice.

In conclusion, the point and purpose of this book is to open a door for you. I'm not trying to give you definitive answers; I'm offering you different ways of bringing Yoga and Āyurveda together that honour each respective science. This is a way of looking at Yoga through the powerful lens of Āyurveda so as to broaden our understanding of Yoga and enhance the practice. And you can refine how you integrate and use these brilliant Yoga tools.

This is meant to be a beginning or a continuation of your exploration—not an end. For those of you who are inspired, I look forward to reading your books on Āyurvedic Yoga, exploring what you've learned, how you teach it, and why you do it the way you do. Let's continue to collaborate, grow, and inspire each other through these beautiful teachings. Let's turn Yoga into healing medicine using Āyurveda so those who need it can find more balance, peace, and harmony within and create balance, peace, and harmony everywhere. Āyurveda teaches us that we are not separate from nature but an integrated part of the whole system. Where each of us finds balance, peace, and harmony, the whole system gets to experience it.

Enjoy!

With love,
m xo
June 2018

FOR FURTHER READING

Āyurvedic-Yoga Books

Frawley, Dr. David. *Yoga & Ayurveda*. Twin Lakes: Lotus Press, 1999.

Frawley, Dr. David and Summerfield Kozak, Sandra. *Yoga for your Type*. Twin Lakes: Lotus Press, 2001.

Styles, Mukunda. *Ayurvedic Yoga Therapy.* Twin Lakes: Lotus Press, 2007.

Āyurveda References

Brown, Christina. *The Ayurvedic Year.* North Adams: Storey Books, 2002.

Caraka + Sharma, Dr. Ram Karan and Dash, Vaidya Bhagwan (translations & commentaries by). *Caraka Saṃhitā*. Varanasi India: Chowkhamba Press, 2014.

Douillard, Dr. John. *The 3-Season Diet*. New York: Three Rivers Press, 2000.

Kripalu School of Āyurveda. *Kripalu School of Āyurveda – Foundations of Āyurveda Student Manual*. 2012.

Lad, Dr. Vasant. *Ayurveda – The Science of Self-Healing*. Twin Lakes: Lotus Press, 2009.

Lad, Dr. Vasant. *Textbook of Ayurveda Fundamental Principles Volume 1*. Albuquerque: The Ayurvedic Press, 2002.

O'Donnell, Kate. *The Everyday Ayurveda Cookbook*. Boston: Shambhala, 2015.

Svoboda, Dr. Robert. *Prakriti*. Twin Lakes: Lotus Press, 1998.

Vāgbhaṭa + Murthy, K R Srikantha. *Aṣṭāṅga Hṛdayam*. Varanasi India: Chowkhamba Press, 2013.

Vāgbhaṭa + Murthy, K R Srikantha. *Aṣṭāṅga Samgraha*. Varanasi India: Chowkhamba Orientalia, 2013.

Welch, Dr. Claudia. *Balance Your Hormones, Balance Your Life*. Cambridge: Da Capo Press, 2011.

"The Elements and their Attributes." *Vibrational Ayurveda* (website). June 19, 2018. http://vibrationalayurveda.com/new-page-1/.

Yoga References

Ashley-Farrand, Thomas. *Healing Mantras*. New York: Random House, 1999.

Clark, Bernie. *Yinsights*. Vancouver BC, 2007.

Gran, Gary. "Ayurveda & Mantra, Part 2." *Yoga Chicago* (website). July 13, 2018. http://yogachicago.com/2014/03/ayurveda-mantra-part-2/.

LePage, Joseph & Lilian. *Mudras for Healing and Transformation*. Seabastopol: Integrative Yoga Therapy, 2013.

Prabhavananda, Swami and Isherwood, Christopher. *How to Know God: The Yoga Aphorisms of Patanjali*. Hollywood: Vedanta Society, 1981.

Vishvketu, Yogrishi. *Yogasana – The Encyclopedia of Yoga Poses*. San Rafael: Mandala Publishing, 2015.

Yoga Journal (website). March 2018 to June 20, 2018, http://www.yogajournal.com.

Sanskrit References

Bachman, Nicolai. *The Language of Āyurveda*. Canada: Trafford, 2010.

Bachman, Nicolai. *The Language of Yoga*. Boulder: Sounds True, 2004.

RESOURCES FOR CAUTIONS AND CONTRAINDICATIONS

As part of writing *Āyurvedic Yoga*, I reached out to fellow yoga teachers to ask, "What are your go-to resources for cautions and contraindications"? The following list contains what I received in response:

1. My yoga teacher and/or yoga teacher-training manual

2. Experience, knowledge, and intuition

3. Trusted teachers ♡, including:

    - Aadil Palkhivala, http://www.aadil.com/author/
    - Baxter Bell, https://www.baxterbell.com/
    - BKS Iyengar, http://bksiyengar.com/modules/Referen/Books/book.htm
    - Diane Ambrosini, *Instructing Hatha Yoga*, 2nd ed., (Champain: Human Kinetics, 2016).
    - Donna Farhi, https://www.donnafarhi.co.nz/product-category/books/
    - Doug Keller, https://www.doyoga.com/bookstore.html
    - Erich Schiffmann, https://erichschiffmann.com/
    - Esther Myers, https://www.estheryoga.com/products/
    - Judith Lasater, http://www.judithhansonlasater.com/reading/

- Julie Gudmestad, https://www.gudmestadyoga.com/julie_gudmestad
- Leslie Kaminoff, https://yogaanatomy.net/
- Loren Fishman, MD, http://sciatica.org/
- Paul Grilley, http://paulgrilley.com/online-courses/
- Purna Yoga, http://purnayoga.com/
- Ray Long, https://www.bandhayoga.com/
- Richard Miller, PhD, https://www.irest.org/publications/Yoga-Nidra-by-Richard-Miller
- Rodney Yee and Nina Zolotow, *Moving Toward Balance* (Emmaus: Rodale, 2004).
- Susi Hately, https://www.functionalsynergy.com/product-category/books/
- Timothy McCall, MD, http://www.drmccall.com/yoga-as-medicine.html
- TKV Desikachar, *The Heart of Yoga* (Rochester: Inner Traditions, 1995).
- Yoga International (was the Himalayan Institute), https://yogainternational.com/
- Yoga Journal website, https://www.yogajournal.com/
- Yoga U Online website and courses, https://www.yogauonline.com/

In addition to these resources, I would like to offer one more thing: Please consider that *working with students is a conversation.*

As teachers, we know what we know. Hopefully, we also

know that there is a lot we don't know. And with this in mind, I approach each student and each class as a conversation. I ask students questions like:

- "How does this feel?"
- "Is this working for you today?"
- "Are you comfortable?"
- "Check in with your body, breath, emotions, mind, and heart."
- "Tell me more ..."

I don't have to have all the answers in this moment. What I do need is to be open to the feedback of the student about his or her own experience, and for us to explore Yoga together with respect for the messages that the body-mind is sharing.

For me, Yoga isn't really about the poses. With that in mind, if I can create space around how we practice *āsana* in order to connect with some of Yoga's other goals, like an increase in self-awareness and freedom from suffering (aka pain), then these *conversations* are immensely fruitful and, honestly, the point of practice.

BIBLIOGRAPHY

"Big." Google. Accessed March 2018. https://www.google.ca/search?q=Dictionary.

Brown, Christina. *The Ayurvedic Year*. North Adams: Storey Books, 2002.

Chödrön, Pema. *Getting Unstuck*. Sounds True, 2005.

Clark, Bernie. *Yinsights*. Vancouver BC, 2007.

"Clear." Google. Accessed March 2018. https://www.google.ca/search?q=Dictionary.

"Cloudy." Google. Accessed March 2018. https://www.google.ca/search?q=Dictionary.

"Cold." Google. Accessed March 2018. https://www.google.ca/search?q=Dictionary.

"Dense." Google. Accessed March 2018. https://www.google.ca/search?q=Dictionary.

Devi, Nischala. *The Secret Power of Yoga*. New York: Three Rivers Press, 2007.

"Dilution." Google. Accessed March 2018. https://www.google.ca/search?q=Dictionary.

Douillard, Dr. John. *The 3-Season Diet*. New York: Three Rivers Press, 2000.

"Dry." Google. Accessed March 2018. https://www.google.ca/search?q=Dictionary.

"Dull." Google. Accessed March 2018, https://www.google.ca/search?q=Dictionary.

Frawley, Dr. David. *Yoga & Ayurveda*. Twin Lakes: Lotus Press, 1999.

Gran, Gary. "Ayurveda & Mantra, Part 2." *Yoga Chicago* (website). July 13, 2018. http://yogachicago.com/2014/03/ayurveda-mantra-part-2/.

"Gross." Google. Accessed March 2018. https://www.google.ca/search?q=Dictionary.

"Hard." Google. Accessed March 2018. https://www.google.ca/search?q=Dictionary.

"Heavy." Google. Accessed March 2018. https://www.google.ca/search?q=Dictionary.

"Hot." Google. Accessed March 2018. https://www.google.ca/search?q=Dictionary.

"Light." Google. Accessed March 2018, https://www.google.ca/search?q=Dictionary.

"Liquid." Google. Accessed March 2018. https://www.google.ca/search?q=Dictionary.

"Mobile." Google. Accessed March 2018. https://www.google.ca/search?q=Dictionary.

"Obvious." Google. Accessed March 2018. https://www.google.ca/search?q=Dictionary.

"Oily." Google. Accessed March 2018. https://www.google.ca/search?q=Dictionary.

"Penetrating." Google. Accessed March 2018. https://www.google.ca/search?q=Dictionary.

Powers, Sarah. *Insight Yoga DVD*. Pranamaya Inc., 2005.

"Rough." Google. Accessed March 2018. https://www.google.ca/search?q=Dictionary.

Sharma, Dr. Ram Karan and Vaidya Bhagwan Dash (translations & commentaries by), *Caraka Saṃhitā* (Varanasi India: Chowkhamba Press, 2014).

"Sharp." Google. Accessed March 2018. https://www.google.ca/search?q=Dictionary.

"Slimy." Google. Accessed March 2018. https://www.google.ca/search?q=Dictionary.

"Slow." Google. Accessed March 2018, https://www.google.ca/search?q=Dictionary.

"Smooth." Google. Accessed March 2018. https://www.google.ca/search?q=Dictionary.

"Soft." Google. Accessed March 2018. https://www.google.ca/search?q=Dictionary.

"Stable." Google. Accessed March 2018. https://www.google.ca/search?q=Dictionary.

"Sticky." Google. Accessed March 2018. https://www.google.ca/search?q=Dictionary.

"Subtle." Google. Accessed March 2018. https://www.google.ca/search?q=Dictionary.

Swami Prabhavananda and Christopher Isherwood. *How to Know God: The Yoga Aphorisms of Patanjali*. Hollywood: Vedanta Society, 1981.

"The densest objects in the universe." ESA. Updated Oct. 15, 2002. http://www.esa.int/Our_Activities/Space_Science/Integral/The_densest_objects_in_the_Universe.

Working Minds. "Quotations from Albert Einstein." Accessed Sept. 4, 2018. https://www.working-minds.com/AEquotes.htm.

GRATITUDE

To Gummo, who sat and talked through Guṇa Yoga with me for HOURS! Who read and re-read. Who encouraged, supported, and helped so much.

To V, who Skypes with me to keep me on track. Who fielded an infinite number of text messages like "What is a sticky *prāṇāyāma*?" And who is always there—my soul twin. I will learn to love the Oxford comma. That's what she said.

To Susan Young, who offered to host a group of my friends to help me figure out what I should write my first book on. Look what you did, Susan! You launched this whole process.

To Laurel, Kathy, and Gummo for joining Susan and me at the meeting—thank you for sharing all your insights and ideas. And thank you, Laurel, for cutting right to the chase with Guṇa Yoga.

To my round-one proofreaders: Sheila, Josh, Gummo, V, Kathy, and Susan. Your feedback made the book so much better! It also made me laugh and smile. Thank you for making the most vulnerable part of this process safe and loving for me.

To Laurel and Kathy, who have proofread everything I have ever written. For your friendship, studentship, and so much support over the past decade.

To Dr. Sonya, who offered thoughtful suggestions, the idea of taking an online how-to-write-a-book course (OMGosh it helped me figure out so much!), and your ongoing support.

To Sarah K, who met me every two weeks to keep me on track. Who feels what is working for me and isn't. Who loves me enough to tell me both these things in a loving and supportive way. Who shakes with me, who cries with me, who laughs like crazy with me.

To Larissa, my Āyurvedic Yoga teacher, who taught me, inspired me, and wouldn't let me get away with being less than I am. Even as it pertained to this project. I am grateful for your presence and honesty in my life. Thank you for being there, for seeing me, for being a true teacher.

To my Āyurveda teachers, Dr. Anusha, Dr. Rosy, Dr. Claudia, Dr. Margrit, Dr. Scott, Dr. Satyanarayan Dasa, Dr. John, Dr. Jyothi, Dr. Lad, Dr. Joshi, Dr. Svoboda, and Dr. Frawley (the last two I have not met, yet I hold them in incredibly high regard and hope to meet them someday). Thank you for sharing your Āyurvedic wisdom. I hope I honoured what you shared and taught. That was my intention.

To my Yoga teachers, Siobhan, Susi, Vishva, Pandiji, Sandy, Richard M, Paul G, Mary C, DC, Mick G, Devarshi, Sudha, and Leslie K. Thank you for inviting me to understand more deeply, for sharing your wisdom, and for reminding me to share the teachings with integrity from my heart.

To my one and only Buddhist meditation teacher, Larry. Thank you. I miss you—a lot.

To my students, who want to learn Yoga and Āyurveda, and who inspire me to want to teach it better. Thank you for showing up. Without you, class is very boring.

To Leela and Ramneek: thank you for your amazing insights into bias, and your support in navigating this aspect of my teaching and writing.

To the team at Janati Yoga School: Thank you for your love and support. I love that we are Janatians. ♡

To the team at Archangel Ink for helping this book be the best and most useful it can be. Kristie Lynn, Rob, Vanessa, Paige, and everyone else: I am grateful for your care and expertise. And your patience when I freak out. Kristie Lynn, thank you for the many ledges you talked me down from.

To my parents, who have supported everything I've ever done for my whole life. Thank you for loving me no matter what. I noticed. It matters. I love you back, no matter what.

To my husband, Glenn, who has been my sounding board and sanity check on this journey of technology, unemployment, Yoga, Āyurveda, and now authorship. Who is the love of my life, my best friend, and my home. I love you. Thank you is not enough for all you do, yet they are the only words I have.

To the Vedas and sages, thank you for these teachings. They have changed my life and made me a better person. I am eternally grateful for your existence and to live in a time when I have access to these rich lessons. *OM*.

ONLINE RESOURCES

Obviously, I'm into Āyurvedic Yoga. As a result, my website (http://www.janatiyoga.com) has lots of different opportunities for you to explore further:

- Free Introduction to Āyurveda Online course
- Āyurveda Basics for Yogis Online course (part of our 300-hr YTT)
- More Āyurveda for Yogis Online (part of our 300-hr YTT)
- Fall 9-day Digestive Reset Program Online (available only in the fall)
- Spring 1-month Digestive Reset Program Online (available only in the spring)
- Postpartum Āyurvedic Self-Care for Mama Online
- Āyurvedic Yoga video classes (doṣic, yin, *agni*, *ojas*, *sattva*)
- Āyurvedic Yoga audio classes

As a thank you for reading the book this far, please enjoy this coupon code for 15% off any audio or video classes from the website: **AYbook15**.

I also run trainings in **Guṇa Yoga** and **Doṣa Yoga** as part of our 300-hr Yoga Teacher Training program. Check our website for dates—it would be great to have you. Or if you have a group that wants to learn more about Āyurvedic Yoga, I can come to you (my *vāta* and the love of my life love to travel!).

A HUMBLE REQUEST

If you enjoyed this book and learned something from it, it would be amazing if you could share your thoughts on Amazon or send me an email. Your honest and sincere review will help others who would benefit from this information to find it more easily. My publishers tell me that it helps more than I can understand.

Thank you for considering.

ABOUT THE AUTHOR

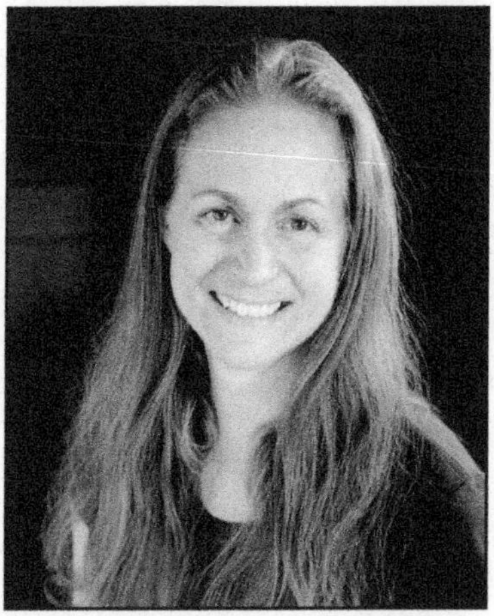

Mona Warner is a warm and joyful educator. Her depth of knowledge, passion, and dedication to the practices of Yoga and Āyurveda are evident. Mona leads by example, and as a student you are encouraged to be and honour yourself, your practice, and others.

Mona works at the Janati Yoga School in Kingston, Ontario, Canada where she lives with her wonderful husband, enthusiastic dog, and ninja kitten. She has been practicing Yoga since 2001, teaching Yoga since 2004, and teaching Āyurveda since 2013. She is a Registered Yoga Teacher Trainer with the Yoga Alliance (ERYT500), a National Āyurvedic Medical Association (NAMA) recognized Āyurvedic Yoga Therapist, and Certified Āyurvedic Practitioner.

When she's not teaching, practicing, or talking about Vedic Sciences, you might find her eating chocolate, reading a book on a beach, climbing a mountain in Ireland, kayaking up to glaciers in Alaska, or zip lining in Costa Rica.